DR. SHANNON
KNOWS

...The 12 STEPS for
WELLTHY
PEOPLE

How To Make **HEALTHY** Your Habit

DR. SHANNON SUBRAMANIAM

Dr. Shannon Knows
© 2011 by Dr. Shannon Subramaniam

Published by Insight Publishing Group
4739 E. 91st Street, Suite 210
Tulsa, OK 74137
918-493-1718

Unless otherwise noted all Scripture quotations are taken from the New International Version, © 1973, 1978, 1984 by The International Bible Society. Used by permission of Zondervan Bible Publishers.

Scripture quotations marked NLT are taken from the Holy Bible, New Living Translation, © 1996, 2004. Used by permission of Tyndale House Publishers, Inc., Carol Stream, Illinois 60188. All rights reserved.

Scripture quotations marked NKJV are taken from the Holy Bible, New King James Version, © 1979, 1980, 1982 by Thomas Nelson, Inc., Publishers.

Cover design by 1260 Productions, www.1260productions.com.

ISBN: 978-1-932503-98-2

Library of Congress catalog card number: 2011930040

Printed in Canada

Here's what leaders are saying about Dr. Shannon and her book:

"This book is a must read for anyone who is trying to maximize their life. Sometimes we all need a kick in the butt to put us on the right path. Dr. Shannon lets you know that there is a way to be your best both mentally and physically. This book makes me want to be a better person. Thank you for the inspiration."

—Bo Van Pelt
PGA Tour Professional Golfer

"Dr. Shannon writes from the heart with the passion of a true believer. If you're ready to make the most of every day you have on this planet, this is the book for you. It will inspire you. It will give you new insight. It will change your life!"

—Terry Hood
CBS News Anchor

"One thing is for certain, Dr. Shannon knows! And now, you will too. I've read this book from cover to cover and been a patient of hers for more than a year. This book will help you from head to toe, and from the inside out. Without hesitation, I fully recommend her words and her care."

—John Mason
Author of numerous best-selling books, including
An Enemy Called Average

"This book contains timeless wisdom, contemporary insights and practical principles, all from a true servant's heart...Dr. Shannon not only shows us *how* to live our best and healthiest lives, but she also inspires us to develop the *desire* to do so. Thank you, Dr. Shannon, for bringing this gift to the world!"

—Dr. David Ajibade
Cofounder and CEO, Building Strength, LLC

"Dr. Shannon knows athletes. She plays an integral role in my approach to a healthy, professional golf lifestyle. She genuinely cares for people's well-being, and I consider her an invaluable part of my team. If you want to discover how to live a healthy life, then I recommend you read Dr. Shannon's book!"

—Greg Mason
Professional Golfer

"In a world that continually sidetracks our lives with 'get-rich-quick, fast-food-mentality living,' Dr. Shannon provides us with a timely gem! In this practical, step-by-step approach to getting *wellthy*, she lays out a strategy that will literally transform your life and get you back on the road to health."

—Dr. Pete Sulack
United Nations Ambassador
Matthew 10 Ministries International Founder
Exodus Chiropractic Founder

"Wow! Dr. Shannon is on a mission to bring this message of health to the world. Her passionate message will motivate and inspire you to take control of your health and get the most out of life. Most importantly, you will walk away with a game plan to transform your life from the inside out! This book is a must read if you are serious about your health and ready to live the life that you were born to live."

—Jonathan Conneely, aka "Coach JC"
Author of *The Secret to Real Weight Loss Success*

"Dr. Shannon was one of my first students whom I taught to use Afformations—empowering questions that change your life. She has not only used Afformations to meet the man of her dreams, she increased her income, got a new office space, and was even given a new car! (You'll learn all about it in chapter 7.) Use this book to become happier and healthier in all aspects of your life. And keep afforming!"

—Noah St. John
Inventor of Afformations
#1 best-selling author of *The Secret Code of Success*

"Dr. Shannon knows! Thank you, Dr. Shannon, for answers about how to live and not just exist. Your twelve steps are very powerful, and the way you have presented them makes perfect sense in our path to being *wellthy*. Having you as a friend has been a great blessing, and now I understand where you get that power of life in your presence! I'm quite sure that the answers people are looking for are between the covers of this book. *Dr. Shannon Knows*—simple but profound solutions."

—Dr. J. Tony Slay
CEO, Ministry International Inc.
President, Ministry International Institute

This book is dedicated to those who seek to know their wellth!

Contents

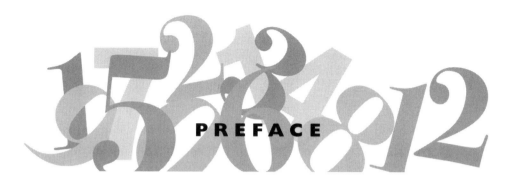

PREFACE

If you're like me, you probably like to skip the preface and get to what you consider as the stuff that really matters. Not this time! I put a lot of important stuff that really matters in the preface you are about to read... Read this and you will be ready, as I was, to take the necessary steps to become healthy and wellthy... This is how to make healthy your habit!

Several years ago, a friend of mine invited me to attend a meeting to hear a person he described as "a great speaker" who was going to share what he referred to as "the best story!" How could I resist? "The best" of anything is incredibly compelling!

We arrived to a packed parking lot and a full meeting room. A young lady stood in front and began to tell her story. I didn't realize then that her story would not only change my life, but would inspire this book—a book that has the power to change your life, too.

She began her story by making a very bold statement that spoke volumes to me; something on the inside of me jumped because her words resonated with my purpose.

The young woman stood in front of hundreds of people and said, "My drug problem started when I was a baby. From antibiotics to antidepressants, every time I had a sniffle, sneeze, or sigh, my parents were putting drugs in my mouth to take my pains away. When I got into high school and college and felt pain, whether physical or emotional, of course I turned to drugs to medicate my hurts. What would you expect me to do?"

After her amazing story of discovering truth and desiring a life of freedom, there wasn't a dry eye in the place. Through my tear-filled eyes, I saw hundreds of people seeking the same thing—a life of freedom. I wanted freedom, even though I had never experienced a drug or alcohol addiction! (Little did I know that while I was writing this book someone very close to me would become addicted to prescription drugs—imagine that... Witnessing the pain and destruction of it firsthand only fueled my passion for this message, and my desire for all of us to live with freedom from whatever it is that is holding us captive.) I was suddenly on a mission to learn more about the 12-Step Program she had talked about, and to find out how it worked. I began to ask questions—lots of them.

To my surprise, two of the three people I was sitting beside had been through the 12-Step Program of Narcotics Anonymous while undergoing treatment for past substance abuse. I listened as one of them described the steps and the group meetings that had helped her immensely in the process. She also explained how they gave her the empowerment, support, and encouragement she needed to walk through the process with her husband. I listened with interest as her husband talked about the 12-Step Program and how he actually "works the steps" daily to continue to remain in recovery; free from drugs and alcohol, clean and sober.

It sounded to me as though this couple's group offered positive, profound empowerment and acceptance. I wondered if I could be a part of such a group, even though I wasn't addicted to drugs or alcohol. I wondered what it would be like to live a life of freedom and have the *best*

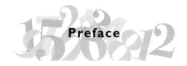

story to tell. I wondered what it would be like to be the *best Shannon* I could be.

I wonder as I wonder...

Have you ever noticed how "wonder" plays a primary role in the beginning of every great thing (including the fact that you are holding this book in your hands and that you're actually reading it)? Reading a book automatically puts you in the top 30 percent of everyone who has ever bought a book. But if you're satisfied with being the top 30 percent of anything, then you may not be ready for these steps. *I'm serious!*

With all due respect, if you're not ready to be your best, give this book to someone who is. You see, so often people are satisfied with just being better; better than they used to be or better than someone else. But "better" or "better than" is not *best*. In fact, I'm going to say that better is an enemy of best, and, in my opinion, is not acceptable. What are *you* willing to accept? *I want to be my best Bailey!*

I believe you picked up this book because you're seeking. Maybe your life seems good, you seem happy, and you think you are healthy, but for some reason, something inside of you is wondering: Could there be more? Am I missing something? Is this all there is?

You're not alone; I've wondered as well!

One day I was wondering what it would be like to be the best in the world at something after watching an inspirational and compelling video about the Women's 1999 World Cup Soccer Team. They had become the best in the world because they dared to wonder what it would be like to be the best (and then they decided to do just that)!

I began to wonder about what the word "wonder" really means. When I looked in the dictionary, these are the definitions I found: "1. a cause of astonishment or surprise : MARVEL...MIRACLE 2. the quality of exciting wonder 3. a feeling...aroused by something extraordinary or affecting."[1]

So if you're excitedly wondering if there's more, then let me assure you, there certainly is more for you! I challenge you to be the *best* in the world at something. What could that be? How about being the *best you* on the entire planet? How about *giving it all*, so when you lie down on your last day on earth, you have absolutely nothing left to give? How about playing this game of life like it's the last game you'll ever play? Why not? *I dare you!*

Looking your best

Best doesn't mean comparing yourself to anyone else, including your *self. Best is about today, right now.* It has everything to do with what your best looks like in this moment. Some days your best may mean being #1 in the world at something, but some days it may mean just being able to get up out of bed and take a shower. What does your best look like today?

Now that I've got you thinking and wondering, let's get back to how this book went from a state of wonder, to a question, to an answer—the answer to so many great and compelling questions. (By the way, thanks for asking these questions and thanks for wondering with me.)

Twelve steps for health

"So if these steps are so profound, why isn't there a 12-Step Program for healthy people to keep them that way?" I asked myself, after hearing that great speaker. Then I asked my friends, but they didn't have the answer either. I reasoned, people usually don't seek such a process unless they have a problem or at least recognize the possibility of something more.

This common mentality sounds dangerously similar to our modern-day "health-care system" in America. Let's face it, the philosophies of "if you feel good, you must be good" and "if it's not broke, don't fix it" just aren't working! According to a 2008 report, America had the most deaths due to preventable diseases, (ranking nineteenth), compared with eighteen

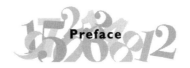
other industrialized nations.[2] According to a Commonwealth Fund report issued in 2008, "101,000 deaths from 2002 to 2003 could have been avoided…"[3] These individuals were someone's loved ones, perhaps one of yours. If so, you have my sincere sympathy. And if not, what if someone had been? What if that someone had been you?

Can you imagine if the only time you took your vehicle in for a checkup was when the red light came on? Of course, you would never do such a thing because you are much more intelligent than that! Did you know that pain in your body is the equivalent of a red light coming on in your car?

Could complacency or being content with "better than" be as danger-ous as denial or a drug addiction? (And perhaps the addiction is to the drugs that are being prescribed every day in America, all in the name of "health"!) Could complacency or contentment with "better than" be what's causing the denial and addictions in the first place?

In light of this complacent mentality, I wondered if people would enroll in a 12-Step Program for healthy people if it were available? Why can't healthy people have twelve steps to keep us functioning well, recov-ered, restored, alive, healthy, and *wellthy*? (Don't worry; I'll define this word soon!) What is available for those of us who want to be "high on life"—who want to get the most out of it, put the most into it, and live life to its fullest?

These were just a few of the questions that came to mind after that first question of what it would be like to be the best, and then came more. I asked, "Why does it have to be drug or alcohol abuse that leads people to the revelation that their lives have become unmanageable and that a power greater than themselves can restore them to sanity?"[4] Could people come to this conclusion without these addictions?

Imagine what 12 Steps for healthy, *wellthy* people to remain healthy and *wellthy* would be like? I did! I envisioned what this "recovery" program would look like.

"Recovery" is: "1. to get back again : REGAIN, RETRIEVE. 2. to regain normal health, poise, or status. 3. to make up for : RECOUP 4. RECLAIM 5. to obtain a legal judgment in one's favor."[5]

Could there be something for someone who hasn't lost anything or had the need "to make up for"? Or even if they had lost something, what if they didn't want to get back only what they'd lost, but so much more? What if they didn't want "normal health," because normal health in our country is, unfortunately, very unhealthy?

My heart and mind kept asking these kinds of questions, and I continued to imagine the incredible possibilities!

Perhaps someone could create "success groups" (I like the sound of that better than "support groups") with weekly huddles (I like the sound of that better than "meetings") for those who were "walking out" the steps instead of "working" them. Imagine if no one had to "work the program," but instead just "lived it" through the unconditional love and possibility of God, themselves, and those who shared a like mind. I was starting to get excited, because I liked the sound of such a concept.

In these groups, what would the atmosphere feel like? I imagined that people would no longer be anonymous. They would *know* who they are, and others would *know* them as well. Members could share themselves and the gifts they'd been given with others, because they would realize that they are blessed to be a blessing.

Where would they meet? "Maybe such a place already existed," I thought. A church, perhaps? Maybe this could be the place to "huddle." Perhaps this would be the place where everyone supported, encouraged, and brought out each other's best. Perhaps; but this was unlike most of the churches I had ever known or experienced.

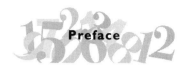

I contemplated some more. Could this "place" actually be a group that trains together several times a week? (Let's face it, for those who really live the program, once a week just wouldn't seem to be enough.)

Then I concluded, what if this place was all of the above, but above all, was *your* place, the place where *you* fit? And what if it wasn't a program at all, but a very familiar place, *and this place was your life*?

Imagine if, by walking the steps, you could actually live the life that you were designed to live. What if you and I could live health (and *wellth*)...for life...for a lifetime? *What if?*

What if you were as healthy as you could be right now? What would that look like? What would *you* look like? How would this affect the rest of your life and the people in it?

What is *wellth*?

So where did all of these questions lead me? To a revelation of something I've coined "*wellth*."

You may be asking yourself, "What in the world is *wellth*?" Or worse yet, you may be thinking it's simply a typo. I assure you that it isn't; in fact, it's very intentional.

Health encompasses so much more than your body, and wealth encompasses so much more than money. True health and wealth can be summed up in one word—*wellth*. Wellth is "the wealth on the inside of you being fully expressed in your body, mind, spirit, and life—it is you at your *best! Your* wellth *is the source of your health!* (For this and more definitions you can go to *Dr. Shannon's Defining Truths* in the back of the book.)

Let me explain...

Stay with me here as I take you on a short *definition tour.* "Wealth" is defined as "1. abundance of possessions or resources 2. abundant supply 3. all property that has a money or an exchange value; also: all objects or resources that have an economic value."[6] The word "wealth" comes from the root word "weal," which means "well-being or prosperity."[7] Now, what is "well"? "Well" is used to describe "best" and "best" is a superlative of "good," which means: "1. of a favorable character or tendency 2. BOUNTIFUL, FERTILE 3. ATTRACTIVE 4. SUITABLE, FIT 5. SOUND, WHOLE 6. AGREEABLE, PLEASANT 7. WHOLESOME 8. CONSIDERABLE, AMPLE 9. FULL 10. WELL-ROUNDED 11. TRUE 12. legally valid or effectual 13. ADEQUATE, SATISFACTORY...COMMENDABLE, VIRTUOUS, KIND."[8]

As I said, another word for "best" is "well." Think about that! "Well" is defined with words such as: "in a good or proper manner: RIGHTLY, EXCELLENTLY, SKILLFULLY, SATISFACTORILY, FORTUNATELY, ABUNDANTLY, COMPLETELY, FULLY, PROSPEROUS, and HEALTHY, or free or recovered from ill health."[9] I love this! Does it make you desire to be well, or what?

When I first got this revelation of the definition of *wellth*, I began speaking to groups big and small about "Creating Health and *Wellth* While on the Move." You see, *wellth* is dynamic; it's ever moving, growing, and changing, just like you and me!

You are your greatest asset! So many people deny their own wellness in pursuit of this or that financial gain, not realizing that if they first and foremost cared for their greatest asset, the return on their investment would be a wealth of health, and a very healthy wealth.

So often, we as humans give up our health for wealth when we're young, only to have to give up our wealth for our health when we get older. Unfortunately, many times there isn't a wealth great enough to buy back the health that we so desperately desire. Then what?

But there's another way, a better way—in my opinion, the *best* way. *The best way is living a life of passionate momentum that creates the powerful blend of health and wealth (wellth) that doesn't trade one for the other, but is the essence of the best of both.*

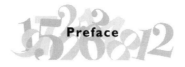

Mission possible

I am on a mission!

This message has awakened me in the middle of the night and in the early hours of the morning. It has kept me awake many a night.

Why? This is a message that will move you from better to best, inspire you on your way to where you're going, and energize you to be the principled, precise, passionate, powerful person you were designed to be. That is exactly what it has done, and is still doing for me.

I believe that you and your generation are in desperate need of, and ready for, something healthier than normal, something more stunning than usual, and something that is uniquely significant. And I believe that you are ready to contribute, not only to your own life, but to the lives of those you touch!

From the title of this book, I may appear to believe I have all the answers, that I *know it all*. I do not know everything, but what I know is this: People do not know that they do not know.

I'm here to help you know what you do not know, and to help you know what you need to know so that you experience whatever it is you're seeking— freedom, healing, weight loss, increased strength, abundance, peace, prosperity, *wellth*, happiness, or health for your life…for your lifetime!

I believe I have a message that everyone can benefit from, but not everyone may be ready to receive. Like a radio, the sound waves may be there, but if the receiver isn't plugged in, the message will pass right by.

Perhaps you *think* you're healthy; you have a great life, a fulfilling existence, a compelling future. Are you willing to *know*? You may be thinking, "Of course I'm willing to know," when perhaps you may not truly be ready to know.

Can you handle the truth? *Imagine if you did…*

I want you to go beyond healing, to a life of *wellth* that will come once you discover the truth, know the truth, speak the truth, and live it with all your heart.

Thinking comes from your head, but knowing comes from your heart. Full expression of life is not lived in our heads, but from above, down, inside, and out! This book contains life-changing information with the ability to transform you in just that way—from above, down, inside, and out. This is what I *know*!

I desire for you to *know* your *wellth*! The only things worse than being unhealthy are (1) being healthy but not *knowing* it; (2) being unhealthy and thinking that you're healthy; and (3) being seemingly stuck in what is, while innately knowing there is *more*! The good news is, freedom is waiting beyond the limits that happen to be embracing you. This is what I desire for all of us, for our entire lifetime.

Are you ready to *know* your *wellth*? Are you ready to know the *well* within you that is the source of all health and prosperity in your life? This is what makes you *wellthy*!

Welcome to your 12 Steps

You're holding the result of asking a series of questions throughout the past few years. As you now know, I asked the first question after hearing that dynamic, courageous young lady tell her inspiring story of how she overcame her life-threatening drug addiction.

We all have a story. It's why we do what we do. To some degree it makes us who we are, up until this point in our lives. Maybe you're seeking answers to the same questions I asked, or maybe you're still trying to decide if this book contains the answers to the questions you've been asking yourself.

I invite you to find out.

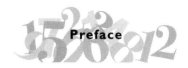

This isn't just "another" 12-Step Program; instead, it is *The* 12 Steps *for* Wellthy *People* to discover the one or more steps they haven't fully taken that will revolutionize their journey of health (and *wellth*)—for life!

Actually, it's *your* first step in the direction your heart is leading you. No, I take that back. It's your second step. Your first step was your desire for something more, which led you to pick up this book in the first place.

God knows how many steps it has taken you to get to this moment— right here, right now! And only you and God will know how many steps it will take you to finish what you've started, and to finish strong.

My confident hope is that you will determine right now to finish the next step, which is to read this book. The most important—crucial, critical, essential, vital—step is that you take Step #12, where you give of yourself and find yourself experiencing health (and *wellth*) for life—for your lifetime!

Everyone loves a great story. I want to help your story be one that is not only great, but one that you will be greatly happy to share.

Thanks for allowing me to share what I know through my "12 Steps." I am still walking them out, and will continue to walk forward in this journey called health…for life!

This is what I know…this is my story!

WELL…come to what I *know*,

Dr. Shannon

GIVING THANKS!

My heartfelt thanks to God! Thanks for being number one in my life and for choosing me to be a messenger. I am honored and feel very grateful "to know." I love and appreciate you!

For my life experiences, especially the hard ones that have given me just enough insight to ask the questions that led to the writing of this book. I thank God for all the lessons I have learned along the way!

To my incredible husband and best friend, Seelan. Thank you for helping me be my best, and loving me even when I'm not. Thank you for believing in me! I have learned so much about success from watching you. Thank you for being *my* captive audience. You are my hero, and I love and respect you more than words can say!

To my wonderful, beautiful, and amazing daughter, Anni. I love and appreciate you so very much! Thank you for making me who I am today. Being your mom is the greatest gift and honor I have ever been given! You are so incredible—I want to be like you when I grow up!

To my two new daughters, Sarah and Michelle. Thank you for adding so much joy to my life, and laughing even when I'm not funny. Thank you for sharing your dad with me, and for completing my family! I love you and am so proud to call you my girls!

To my fabulous parents, for raising me with a healthy lifestyle, even before it was cool to take vitamins and drink bottled water! Thank you for being one of the few constants in my life and always being there and loving me for who I am! I love and appreciate you so very much!

To my dear and best friend, Dr. Mel (lovingly known as "Melly" ☺). Wow, where would I be without you? You know me so well; better than I know myself at times. Thank you for that, and thank you for always sharing what you know with me. Thank you for keeping me accountable to who I am—and the truth. Thanks for being there every step of the way. I love you, girl!

To my awesome coach and friend, John Mason, from Insight Publishing Group. Wow! We did it! Thank you for all your wisdom, insight, and help in communicating this message to the world. Your powerful expertise has challenged me to truly go deeper and further than I thought I could. Just when I thought I was done, you helped me see that I was just beginning. Thank you for believing in me and the message. Thank you for being healthy and *wellthy*!

To Linda Mason. You are such a ray of sunshine! Thank you for taking my message and putting it into a format that people can read and understand. You are the greatest editor and encourager. Thank you for asking me the tough questions and for noticing every answer and every last word! Thank you for being bold, and asking, "Why?" You have challenged me to discover a new appreciation for all the details—every last one of them! Thank you from the bottom of my heart!

To Dr. Travis, Dr. Tony, Gary, and Kit. Thank you for giving me the title of this book. Thanks for being "in the know" and helping me share it with the world. I will never forget that incredible one-hour-and-forty-minute van ride on May 11 in India! (Yes, Gary, the 11th! ☺) It's because of that journey that you hold what "Dr. Shannon Knows" in your hands.

To Noah St. John. Thanks for giving me (and the world) Afformations! We are so grateful!

To all the past and future *health4life REVOLUTION!* TRANSFORMA-TION CHALLENGE participants. Every year, you challenge and inspire me more than I could ever imagine! Thank you for your commitment, diligence, and decision to be your best and to do "health"…for a lifetime!

To all our past and future *health4life REVOLUTION!* TRANSFOR-MATION CHALLENGE sponsors and partners. Without you, "health4life" would just be a good idea. Thank you so very much for helping it become a REVOLUTION! We are transforming the health and *wellth* of those in our community and around the globe. Thank you for making it possible!

To my mentor and friend, Dr. Pete, for opening up a gateway to fulfilling a deep dream and calling of mine—India! Thank you for being such a remarkable leader and life changer. You inspire me! Thank you for being the powerful leader that you are in our most awesome profession!

To my mentors and friends, Dr. Schiffman and Mama Vicki. Thank you for showing me that it *is* possible, and for never giving up on me on my way through what seemed like the impossible! For doing what's never been done before in the history of chiropractic, and caring enough about people to show others how to do greater things than even you have done. For your unwavering integrity, faith, and commitment, and for always being faithful and *all in*! I love and appreciate you!

To yet another mentor, coach, and friend, Dr. Braile. Thanks for being who you are and for all you've done in keeping chiropractic alive and well! I appreciate you!

To Dr. Jim Richards, for helping me rewrite truth on my heart!

To Kelli Crawford. Thanks for your incredible transcription skills!

To Aspen and Josh with 1260 Productions. This book wouldn't have made it without you! *I* wouldn't have made it without you. Your creativity and innovation, as well as flexibility and friendship, are such a blessing to me. Thank you for your amazing talents and your incredible patience! You guys are the very best! (www.1260productions.com)

To all my dear and faithful patients over the years (and for the next seventy years! ☺). You are why I am right here, right now. You are why I do what I do! Thank you for inspiring me to continue to be the best that I can be—the healthiest, *wellthiest,* happiest doctor (which means teacher) possible. I am committed to doing everything I can to help you be your best and live health and *wellth* for a lifetime! Thanks so much for your commitment, your trust, your support, your amazing referrals, and for being healthy/*wellthy* role models for the world to appreciate. Please know that I appreciate and love each and every one of you!

To all of my beautiful, precious girls (widows and orphans) in India, for touching my heart in such a way that now I know more than ever why I wrote this book and why I am here!

To each of you, my readers! You are the ones I wrote this book for. I saw some of your faces as I wrote this (you know who you are ☺). Thank you for purchasing this book and investing in your *wellth* by taking the steps necessary for health and *wellth* for life. Thank you for sharing your steps with me, and thanks for sharing in my steps and making it all worth it! Thank you for *knowing* your *wellth,* prospering in health, and helping others do the same. Together, we can make the world a healthier, *wellthier* family!

Finally, to everyone who has already said great things about this book, as well as those of you who will, *thank you so much*!

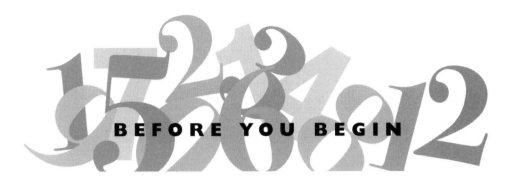

BEFORE YOU BEGIN

Did you know?

Wellth is "the wealth on the inside of you being fully expressed in your body, mind, spirit, and life—it is you at your best! Your wellth is the source of your health!"

Years ago, I knew in my heart that I desired to do mission work in India. I had always been fascinated with the selfless service of Mother Teresa and felt drawn to serve there as well. A few times I had an opportunity to go, but the timing just never seemed right. Finally, after over ten years, I traveled to India to serve with a group of leaders.

After seven unforgettable days of witnessing miracles, signs, and wonders, we loaded our luggage back on a van, and took off on our journey home to the United States. After a week of death-defying driving (or should I say, "riding") experiences, I came to realize two things about Indian transportation: (1) unlike American rules of the road, Indians drive in the left lane; and (2) besides the brakes, the most important part of a van is its horn. The horn seemed essential for saying pretty much every salutation, good-bye, get over, get out of the way, coming through, and four-letter expletives necessary for the typical Indian driver. (Let's just say, the horn had a universal language all its own!) I was just glad that it kept us all alive and well on several occasions.

After seeing that our driver could handle just about anything coming at him, we decided to leave the driving to him, and I, along with each of my colleagues, attempted to summarize our life-changing experience the best way we could with our own limited vocabulary. Words just didn't seem to do any of it justice. But somehow amidst the horn-blowing and the random combination of accelerating, swerving, and braking, we all seemed to understand what the other was trying to say. (I will tell you more about my experience later in the book.)

Then one of my friends said he was going to start eating better and exercising more once he got back to the States. I began to share with him my eating and exercise program and the necessary truths that are vital to living a healthy (*wellthy*) life for a lifetime.

I explained how important a renewed mind-set is to making *healthy* a habit. So many people think that if they want to lose weight, get in great shape, or live a better life that they have to go on a diet, work out, or get more or less of something. Worse yet, they may even think that they're not good enough just the way they are. Instead, it's about knowing the truth and being the best you that you can be, I said.

As I shared what I knew, everyone in the van began to listen in. I pointed out the fact that so many people do not know the truth about who they are, why they're here, and how their bodies are designed to function. I said, "People just don't know. And the most disturbing thing is that many do not even know that they do not know."

That's when I heard the voice of my friend, Dr. Travis, emanating from the back of the van: "But Dr. Shannon knows."

Then another friend, Dr. Tony, enthusiastically encouraged me to share this with others so they could know what they need to know. I told him that I was already doing so, and that I was writing a book about it. Everyone was very excited to hear about my book, but when they heard the title, *The 12 Steps to Health for Life*, they unanimously insisted that it instead be called, *Dr. Shannon Knows* (ultimately becoming, *Dr. Shannon Knows…The* 12 Steps *for* Wellthy *People*—because when you *know* your *wellth*, you can prosper in your health).

I agreed. Not because I know it all, but because this is what I *know* to be true. It has drastically changed my life, and I know that it can do the same for you. That is, if you are willing.

If you're not willing to be your best, then this book is definitely *not* for you! Are you willing to be the answer to the questions you're asking? Imagine if you were the solution to your problems or someone else's? *Did you know that your life is the answer to the questions you've been asking?*

Defining your health

How healthy/*wellthy* are you right now? Is health/*wellth* a relative term or is it an absolute, because it's life? I believe it's life…absolutely! If you are healthier/*wellthier* than you were five years ago, but you're still unhealthy, are you healthy/*wellthy*?

I'm going to ask you three of the most fundamental questions you'll ever answer in regard to your health. Are you ready? (I guess that makes four questions. ☺) Here they are:

1. Are you healthy? *More so than the past, but not the best.*

2. How do you know if you are healthy? *Idk*

3. How do you define health? *How young your spirit is! How young your body (everything) 7 feels & looks*

My experience has shown me that, hands down, how you define health has a bigger influence on your health and how you care for yourself and how you live your life than anything else.

Your definition of health is bigger than all the "good" or even "great" information ever written on the subject. It's more powerful than any "should" you will ever tell yourself or be told by someone in regard to what you "should" do or not be doing to be healthy. Your definitions in life will not only determine your behavior (the message of your life), but the meaning of your life (what that message means to you and others in your life).

If you focus on changing only your behavior and not the source of that behavior, your results will be average and temporary, if that. This is exactly how *not* to be your best!

What if you consciously defined or redefined your definition of health, *wellth*, success, or whatever area in your life needs a tune-up (or tone-up)? What if you allowed your life to become defined? How would that look? How would *you* look? And what would that mean to you?

Step by step in this book, you will see what your defined life looks like. And with each step, you will walk out the life that God has for you.

The Bible says, "For wide is the gate and broad is the road that leads to destruction, and many enter through it. But small is the gate and narrow the road that leads to life, and only few find it."[1] I believe the gate and road are small because you must enter and walk through on your own. But that doesn't mean you have to do it alone because you will follow the One who prepared the way for you and, by doing so, you will lead others in the same direction. You will be making a lasting and significant contribution. You will not only be living a legacy, but leaving one for others to follow.

Step in time

An experience at a training camp in Texas on November 1, 1997, left me with a powerful memory. I was running with two fellow chiropractors just as the sun was setting. My friend had just shared the importance of rhythm and breath while running, and all three of us had gotten into a harmonic cadence in both. (For me, running is metaphorical to life; it's a dynamic masterpiece, and when you find your rhythm, you can enjoy the song of your life with ease. It also reminds me of life because sometimes when I run, it's hard, and I feel like giving up…but because I have found my rhythm and breath…*I do not*! ☺ Once I ran with a friend who had not run before. She kept telling me that she couldn't do it. Then I said, "Yes you can! Even though you may feel like you're going to die, you're not!" She kept going, she found her rhythm and breath, she did not die, *and* she became a runner!) Now back to my story… ☺

All of a sudden, I thought I saw car lights coming toward us from behind, but oddly enough, I couldn't hear anything. The lights were like the intensity of a setting sun. In fact, the sun was almost set so I thought perhaps that's what it was. When I turned to look over my shoulder to see where the light was coming from, there was nothing but a bright glow. I could sense the presence of masses of people, and the energy they were radiating was brilliant, warm, and peaceful. I felt as though God was showing and telling me that this light was from those I would lead. In that moment, I knew it would be masses of people.

What I find most interesting about the timing of that experience was the fact that it happened when there was harmony in rhythm and breath with those I was running with. My question for you is, "Are you ready to move with rhythm and breath in all that God has in store for you?"

If yes, then keep reading. Keep stepping forward as you become the healthiest, *wellthiest* person you can be!

Are you ready to run? If so, then let's go! That running experience in the middle of Texas was truly an unforgettable one—may ours be as well.

Your Health/*Wellth* Locator

Are you willing to discover what you do not know, and "know that you know that you know" exactly what you do know? Then this book is precisely for you—I just know it! YES!

To help prepare you for your first step and to propel you ahead in each successive step, here I have included your "Health/*Wellth* Locator." A *TIME* magazine article entitled "America's Health Checkup" asked the question, "What is the measure of a country's health?" and answered it by stating: "One way is by taking a close look at yourself."[2] To this I proclaim, "I agree!" That is exactly what you and I are going to do…

How Do You Know You Are Healthy/*Wellthy?* (Please answer "Yes" or "No" to *know*)

1. **Are you currently taking any drugs (prescribed, over the counter, or illegal)?** Yes.

   Yes, ibuprofen is a drug. So is aspirin!

   Did you know, in 1996, 7,600 Americans died and 76,000 were hospitalized due to taking Non-Steroidal Anti-Inflammatory Drugs (NSAIDS), which include ibuprofen, aspirin, and naproxen?[3]

   Did you know that prescription drug abuse is up 80 percent in America?[4]

   Whatever happened to "Just say *no* to drugs"? We tell our children this and yet we pop pills into them every time they hurt.

   Every time you take a drug, whether you like it or not, there is a side effect.

   There is no such thing as a safe drug!

   They may be relatively safe, meaning they may be safe for your friend's relative, but may be fatal to yours.

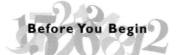

Think twice before you put a drug into your body!

Ask questions; *know* the facts; read the small print…

"Just say KNOW to drugs."

The Centers for Disease Control and Prevention (CDC) issued the fact that in 2007, more than 27,600 Americans died due to unintentional drug poisoning. Prescription pain medications were responsible for half of those deaths.[5]

2. **Are you currently experiencing any pain in your body?** *Yes.*

Pain is not your problem; the cause of your pain is—but pain is a warning signal. You can have a problem and not have pain, but if you have pain, there is something causing that pain.

Find the cause!

3. **Are you able to sleep at night?** *Depends*

Sleep is when your body restores and rejuvenates. If you're not sleeping, you are not rebuilding. If you're breaking down faster than you're rebuilding, you are headed for a breakdown.

Did you know, according to the Institute of Medicine, in 2007, 70 million Americans suffered from insomnia?[6]

In that same year, "Americans spent almost $1.8 billion filling more than 16 million prescriptions for Ambien and Ambien CR."[7]

Did you know that people who have taken Ambien, a medication prescribed to treat insomnia, have experienced side effects such as: "getting out of bed while not being fully awake and doing an activity that [they] do not know [they] are doing" (aka "sleep driving"); "abnormal thoughts and behavior…suicidal thoughts or actions?"[8]

Remember, there is no such thing as a safe drug!

4. **Do you wake up feeling rested and energized?** *Hardly Ever! I'm*

    Many people sleep, but not everyone rests. We were designed to rest, and if we're not resting, we are not functioning according to, or agreeing with, the divine plan (which is to function the way we were designed to function).

    Someone once told me that rest is when we come into agreement with God.

    A lack of agreement causes a lack of rest, and so on, and so on! Imagine the energy you would have if you weren't caught up in this tiresome cycle.

    Did you know that fatigue is one of the first signs of dysfunction in the body? Doesn't it make sense to find out what's causing it, instead of just masking it with a drug?

5. **Are you able to function without caffeine?** *Yes*

    If you continue to substitute unhealthy energy from the outside, in…your body will never have the opportunity to tap into its own natural, healthy energy from above, down, inside, and out.

    (By the way, did you know that caffeine is a drug? Return to question #1.)

    Being fatigued is your body's way of saying, "Help," not "More caffeine, please!"

    Did you know, in 2003, CBS News reported that "50% of Americans drink coffee every day—three to four cups each, more than 330 million cups a day and counting?"[9]

    And when you add other caffeinated drinks, the percentage is closer to "80% of Americans."[10]

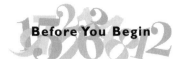

CBSnews.com reported, "Caffeine intoxication is on the rise" and "more and more caffeine abuse victims are showing up in the nation's emergency rooms."[11]

6. **Do you eat fast food?** *Yes ...*

Healing takes time and repetition.

Our bodies weren't constructed in a day, nor do they build and repair in a day.

To do this, they need strong building materials; if you want your life to last as long as it possibly can, give your body the life-giving, life-sustaining food it was designed to live on.

Did you know that Americans spend more than $148.6 billion a year on fast food?[12]

7. **Do you smoke or use tobacco products?** *NO!! el I'm a SWAT member!*

You already know the commentary for this question. "Smoking" is at the top of your "Shouldn't" list, and "Stop smoking" is at the top of your "Should" list.

Every time you light up, you are burning years off your life.

Enough said—when you decide to stop, you will!

8. **Do you eat a lot of dairy products?** *No.*

We are the only species that drinks another species' milk. Just that thought alone is enough to make me question the nature of drinking the milk that a baby cow was designed to drink. You are not a cow!

Dairy products can cause mucus production to increase in the body, which can cause not only congestion, but a whole lot of other symptoms that could easily be put to rest by avoiding, or at least limiting, dairy consumption.

You may suffer from lactose intolerance. Could it be that you're intolerant for a very good reason, and it's not because there is something wrong with you; instead, your body is acting exactly the way it should to keep you healthy?

9. **Do you eat a lot of red meat?** *Yes...*

Eating red meat can cause your body's inner pH balance to become more acidic and imbalanced in nature. This can cause a multitude of symptoms and health concerns.

What do you think of when you hear the words "lactic acid"? That's right, pain.

Is avoidance of acid-causing red meat starting to make sense?

10. **Do you eat a lot of processed food?** *Yes...*

Once again, we were designed to eat life-giving food. What is life-giving food?

It's the kind of food that becomes covered with green stuff if you leave it on your counter for a time. Processed food doesn't sustain life for the "green stuff," so what makes us think it will sustain us?

11. **Do you use artificial sweeteners?** *Nope ... I'm allergic!*

Who wants the knock-off handbag or the Frauda Prada?

Artificial anything is not valuable or healthy, period. Do an Internet search on the negative effects of artificial sweeteners such as aspartame and you will see for yourself.

12. **Do you consume a lot of sugar?** *Yes...*

Let me just say that cancer cells thrive on sugar; healthy cells do not. Which cells do you want to feed and support? *Healthy!!!*

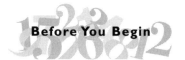

Did you know that the average American consumes 180 pounds of sugar each year?[13]

13. Do you drink soda or ~~sweetened tea?~~ *ou yes!*

Soda and tea can contain caffeine, sugar, and/or artificial sweeteners. Yikes, we have already talked about this! Many sodas also contain phosphoric acid, which causes your body's pH level to become more acidic. When this occurs, the body will leach minerals from your bones to normalize the alkaline pH of your blood. Have you heard of osteoporosis?

Did you know that simply eliminating liquid calories from your diet can allow you to lose weight?

14. Do you take vitamin and mineral supplements daily? *no.*

I would love to tell you that if you eat well, you would get all the vitamins and minerals that you need. But this is simply not true.

The nutrient content of our food depends on the nutrients in the soil. The soil that our food is grown in just does not contain the healthy mineral content that it did years ago. Not to mention all the chemicals, pollutants, and medications that we may be exposed to every day that directly affect our bodies and their ability to absorb the nutrients from the food we eat! Minerals are essential for life.

Dr. Henry Schroeder has so brilliantly stated, "Minerals are the basic spark plugs in the chemistry of life, on which the exchanges of energy in the combustion of foods and the building of living tissues depend." Proper supplementation is essential for optimal function and your best health!

15. Do you eat green vegetables every day? *Usually*

Vegetables, especially the green ones, cause your body's pH to be more alkaline. This has the opposite effect of dairy, red meat, sugar, and sodas. Green vegetables (especially when they're eaten raw) are life-giving, life-sustaining food.

16. Do you have regular daily bowel movements? *yes*

All healthy environments have a way of getting rid of waste and they do it often.

Did you know that 4 million Americans suffer from constipation?[14]

Could it be that we've become a nation of people full of "you know what"? ☺ *BaHahahahahaha!* ☺

17. Do you drink at least half your body weight in ounces of pure water every day? *More like ¼ ... "*

We are primarily water. The more we drink, the more we will be what we were designed to be.

18. Do you eat more than once or twice a day? *Depends.*

If not, you could be slowing down your metabolism, and without a healthy functioning metabolism, your body will store body fat. Your body may be functioning in "starvation" mode and if so, it will go into "storage" mode.

Did you know that this is why a camel has a hump? It is storing up food and water for later.

Do you have some humps you would like to get rid of? *yes!*

19. Do you eat breakfast? *No.*

Someone once told me that sumo wrestlers are not allowed to eat breakfast. I actually researched this and found that it's true. "People

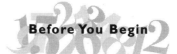

who do not have breakfast, like sumo wrestlers, have a 5% lower metabolism than those who don't skip breakfast."[15]

Have you ever seen a sumo wrestler?

20. Do you exercise at least three times per week, including both cardiovascular and strength training? *Yes,*

Motion is life and life is motion. If you're not moving, you are slowing dying.

The more muscle you have, the greater your metabolism or fat-burning capacity.

21. Do you see a chiropractor at least one to four times a month to be checked for nerve interference? *Yes.*

The power that made the body, heals the body. Our bodies were designed to be self-healing.

Our bodies can heal themselves as long as nothing interferes with that healing.

Vertebral subluxation (spinal misalignment) can cause nerve interference that can lead to less than optimal health. Chiropractors locate and correct nerve interference.

22. Are you truly happy? *I do not believe so.*

(By the way, how do you define happy? ☺)

Happy is healthy! Healthy is *wellthy!*

23. Are you peaceful? *I do not believe so.*

The Bible says that we should let peace be our guide. If there is no peace, what will guide us?

24. Do you love what you do? *Most of the time*
6¾ of 7 days a week

Love never fails.

25. Do your relationships, especially the most intimate ones, bring out your best? *No.*

Our relationships are either adding to or subtracting from us. Do the math.

26. Do you have any grudges or grievances toward anyone in your life right now (including yourself)? *Yes.*

"Forgive, and you will be forgiven."[16]

Forgiveness is healing.

27. Do you believe in a spiritual power higher than yourself? *Yes.*

In the beginning was God, He created all things, and we were made in His image. Therefore, we have the creative power of the universe available to us.

Nothing is impossible!

28. Are your most dominant thoughts during the day positive or negative?

Someone told me, "Thought is cause." I agree—we are what we think about.

Take a look at yourself and your life, and you will have the answer to this question.

29. Are the words you speak predominantly positive or negative?

Our thoughts become our words. We hold the most creative or destructive force imaginable right in our very own heads!

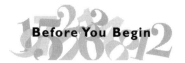

Someone once told me that there are three types of people. There are those who talk about other people; those who speak about places and circumstances; and, those who speak about possibilities and ideas! Which one are you? *1st, but I wana be the 3rd!*

30. **Are you settling for less than your best?** *Yes... But not anymore.*

Anytime we settle, we "...sink gradually to a lower level."[17]

Why would you do that to yourself? Please stop doing that to yourself.

31. **Do you have a plan for being and staying healthy?** *No.*

My patient, Mark, told me this the other day: "If I knew I was going to live this long, I would have taken better care of myself."

Regret is more penetrating than sickness and death.

32. **Are you afraid that you may not be as healthy (and *wellthy*) as you would like to be?** *Yes.*

Fear not—there is *hope*!

As long as life is flowing through you, there is hope for a healthier, *wellthier* tomorrow!

33. **Are you healthy? Are you *wellthy*? Are you willing to be?**
No   no   Yes!

34. **Are you willing to make *healthy* your habit?** *Yes!*

As human beings, we are creatures of habit. If we are going to have a habit, why not make it a healthy one?

If you're thinking that was a lot of questions, you're right, but *within these questions lie profound truths for you.* Your answers will define (or redefine) you, just as the answers to the questions I've asked myself over the

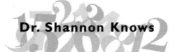

last several years have defined me, what I know, and what I'm about to share with you.

About a year after I asked that famous first question that I wrote about in the preface (when I wondered, "What would it be like to be the best Shannon I could be?"), I was reading the Bible one day and got so inspired that I began to write. I had no idea that as I was writing about what I knew, I was actually beginning to write *The* 12 Steps *for* Wellthy *People*.

And here they are…

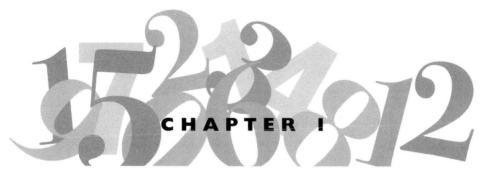

CHAPTER 1

Step #1: Expose Yourself

Did you know?

*When you're afraid, your natural tendency
is to cover up and hide.*

What are you hiding from?

When you're hiding, you'll find it extremely difficult to move forward, or even to move at all! Do you remember playing hide-and-seek as a kid? I was very small, so I always found places to hide that seemed impossible for anyone to find me. The problem was, I was usually stuck in a small, dark place, unable to move. Looking back, I wonder who was winning—the one hiding or the one seeking?

What are you afraid of? Have you ever noticed that you don't run to something you fear, but away from it? For that reason, it might help to uncover what you're afraid of by asking yourself, "What am I running from?"

I used to respond quickly to these questions by saying, "Nothing!" What was disturbing about my answer wasn't even so much in what I said, but in what I thought; I honestly thought I was telling the truth. I soon realized, there is nothing scarier than not knowing the truth and basing personal fearlessness upon it.

So please do yourself a favor; don't respond quickly to my questions. And let me encourage you, if these questions make you feel a little uncomfortable, agitated, nervous, or scared, then there's hope for you.

As a human being, it's easy to think this way of yourself: "I, of all people, shouldn't be afraid of anything, right? I have it all together. I am successful; I'm a mover and a shaker, a leader, and a mother (or a father). I'm the one everyone else comes to when feeling scared or unsure and when needing advice. So how can I be afraid?"

Being afraid isn't our problem, but living in fear is.

The truth is, we all are afraid of something, at some time or another, but even this admission isn't the whole truth. Ironically, being afraid isn't our problem, but living in fear is. Why? Because living in fear smothers, isolates, paralyzes, and eventually suffocates us, suddenly and drastically affecting everyone around us. Take for instance, the times I hid in a small, dark place as a child. If I had never come out of hiding, eventually everyone would have been looking for me and missing out on knowing the person God created me to be. In a case like that, who wins? Neither the one hiding, nor the ones seeking. Everyone loses.

To say you're not afraid of anything is simply not honest. Until you're honest with yourself, you will never be able to take the next step necessary for living a healthy and *wellthy* life! Please note: I rarely use the word "never," but there just doesn't seem to be a word that speaks the truth more simply in this scenario. You'll see for yourself when you get to Step #2.

If you're honestly having a hard time answering what you're afraid of because for many years you've avoided "it" (whatever *it* is for you), let me give you a hint. Take an open look at yourself spiritually, mentally, physically, emotionally, relationally, and financially and answer this question: "In any of these areas, is my life lacking in freedom, abundance, success, fulfillment, health and *wellth?*" Once you identify them, I encourage you to look deeper. Somewhere at the root of your lack is a fear that has caused you to be less than your best—less than healthy, less than *wellthy*.

You finished the previous chapter by asking yourself a lot of questions which, hopefully, began to expose some answers (possibly hidden ones you didn't even know were there). How did you answer the question "Are you afraid you're not as healthy (and *wellthy*) as you would like to be?"

I also asked you how you define health for yourself. When I asked myself this question many years ago (to make a long story short), I answered by saying, "Health is full expression of life." That is my personal definition, although it may not be yours.

What are we afraid of? This question causes us to become truly honest. It causes us to expose our weakness, our vulnerability, and our unhealthiness, and it doesn't feel very comfortable. Feeling this way may cause us not only to cover up, hide, or shrink back, but to ignore what seems to be staring us in the face and to deny the truth. Those reactions are exactly what "full expression of life" is not! In order to experience our full expression of life, we must expose the truth regarding the light and the darkness hidden inside of us.

Naked and unashamed

Several years ago, I fulfilled a lifelong dream of mine when I opened my own fitness studio. (I began teaching fitness classes in 1985 and have loved the thrill and reward of instructing thousands of people ever since!)

Before opening my studio, lots of people questioned me about whether or not I was going to install mirrors on the walls. Some said mirrors would make them feel uncomfortable, while others loved the idea. At the time, many so-called experts in the fitness industry contradicted each other; some saying that mirrors on the wall would have a negative effect on individuals with a poor body image, while others argued the opposite. That controversy left me in a position to decide for myself what was best for my clients.

> ## *"Until you are able to see what is, you will have a very difficult time seeing what can be."*

This is what I decided: naked and unashamed! I told my clients that training in front of mirrors would make it easier for them to stand naked and unashamed in front of their mirrors at home. I told them that, sooner or later, they were going to have to look in their mirrors and see themselves as they were. Through tough love, I told them, "It is what it is, but it doesn't have to stay that way, and it won't. I will help you. Until you are able to see what is, you will have a very difficult time seeing what can be."

The same is true for you. It's time to make a decision, once and for all, to expose your fears and see them for what they are. You can't deal with whatever it is you fear until you expose it. And you can't expose your fears until you're brave enough to expose yourself inside and out—naked and unashamed. You may be thinking, "I can do naked, but it's the unashamed part I have trouble with." Well, we all start somewhere! ☺ When you start facing your fears, you'll discover that "ashamed" will begin to transform into "unashamed," I promise.

Naked and unashamed is the purest form of confronting fear once and for all. It's the best way to put fear in its place, which is exposed outside instead of hidden inside.

I instructed my clients to stop standing in front of their mirrors at home and saying, "I'm not *that* bad!"

"Compared to whom?" I'd ask. "Besides, who wants to be any degree of bad? Telling yourself you don't look too bad is like saying, "Not too bad" when asked, "How are you?" Please neither compare yourself to bad nor to an ideal picture you impose upon yourself.

Instead, stand exposed and say, "It is what it is, so what am I going to do about it?" (No matter what you're revealing to yourself from the inside or the outside.) Have you ever thought about simply giving thanks for what is? (We will discuss this later—when you are ready for Step #5. ☺)

By the way, as you've probably guessed, I chose to put a lot of mirrors on my studio walls. However, I also offered a small mirror-free area for those who weren't quite ready to see for themselves. Not everyone is ready to know the truth. Until people are ready, they cannot move past their fears into joyous, full expression of life.

If you are one of these people, someone who is feeling like you're not quite ready to move ahead, please allow me to encourage you by telling you that it's acceptable to "feel afraid and do it anyway." I think someone once described that as being courageous. And let me once again encourage you by saying, "What is, is not necessarily what will be."

What's missing?

"Is this all there is?" That is one of the scariest questions I have ever asked myself; not because the answer was scary, but because I was shocked to find myself asking it in the first place! You see, I am one of the most positive people around. Those who know me well often call me things like "the shiny side of the coin" and "the happy-maker." I choose to see the glass not just half full, but *full,* so in my mind, I would be the least likely one to ask such a seemingly sad question.

But I believe I'm not the only one who has ever suddenly been confronted with this question. I also believe that I'm not the only one who then asked, "Where did this question come from?" At the time, my life seemingly had all the right ingredients, but somehow something was missing.

A movie I watched as a kid portrayed the story of a group of successful businessmen who came together after years of living in the "real, adult world" only to discover that they were restless, unsatisfied, and unfulfilled.

Some of them even defined themselves as miserable. Something was missing and each of them made the conscious decision to find out just what that "one thing" was.

That *one thing* was calling. A calling is not the same for all of us. It may be just one more piece, another step, or perhaps just a different configuration of the pieces you already have. Through either a minor adjustment or a major correction in focus, suddenly, your picture will become clear.

Asking myself, "Is this all there is?" has certainly changed not only the course of my life, but hopefully will change the course of yours as well. Maybe, just maybe, you've never asked that question. Instead, you've said, "It just doesn't get any better than this!" That's awesome, but what if there is more? What if your good could be great? What if your great could be the greatest? What if your better could be the best? Come on, I dare you to wonder. What are you afraid of?

Expose yourself! Wow, now that's easier said than done…or is it?

Out of step

When I first finished the manuscript of this book, I had this step as Step #2. Then, I woke up one day shortly after with the revelation that until fear is addressed, and you see who you really are underneath all that outside and inside interference, all your steps will be hindered, especially this one. Your steps (your life) will be misaligned by one of the biggest epidemics known to all humans: fear! Did you know that the opposite of love is not hate, but fear? That's right; and when you live in fear, you'll find it not only difficult to love others, but I believe, impossible to truly love at all, especially yourself and the God who created you. God *is* love! Fear is *not*!

Without facing your fear, it's impossible to see who you are and where you really are.

Facing your fear honestly and openly helps you transform fear into faith. How? By reconnecting to your hopes!

What do you hope for today, tomorrow, and the rest of your life? Hope makes your life easier. With ease, dis-ease has no place in your life! This is a chief cornerstone for your foundation for health (and *wellth*)...for life.

Fear doesn't change your future; it creates it.

Fear doesn't change your future; it creates it. Faith changes your future *and* creates it. Therefore, it only makes sense to choose faith in any, and all, circumstances. When you see fear for what it really is—powerless, unless you are led by it—you will be fully able and empowered to take the next step, and the next!

When fear leads you, that which you fear does come upon you; yes, it's true! Whatever we fear will eventually flow out of us, from the inside out, into our lives. Then we will be forced to look at it face-to-face, once and for all. We will then want to blame others or feel sorry for ourselves because of what is happening. The truth is, fear is very lazy and it loves when we do all the work—by the time fear manifests in our lives, we're already worn out from all the stress and strain of carrying it around, hidden inside of us for so long. On top of all that, now we think we're the victim and this makes us feel even more powerless and seemingly unable to fix or rise above our circumstances. In essence, we become walking paralytics.

What makes fear so disabling and the cause of most, if not all, dysfunction is that it is full of endless possibilities of impossibility. What? That's right, because whether we fear something that's real or imagined, it is real to us and becomes our reality. The negative possibilities of fear are limitless. It's absolutely vital for us to learn how to recognize fear and deal with it each time it arises, so we can put an end to it once and for all.

What I've learned about fear is that it truly comes to rob us of our peace, kill our dreams, and steal our future. I have heard fear described in so many ways: "false evidence appearing real" (thank you, Joyce Meyer); "forget everything and run" (I believe this one came from Dr. Jim Richards); and, somewhere I heard, "feel everything and run!" However, no definition of fear will mean more to you than the one you give to it.

Fear is...

Did you know that you—yes, you—get to decide what fear is going to mean to you? That's right! You get to decide not only what it means to you, but also what you're going to do with it; how you will allow it, or not allow it, to affect your life.

When fear comes upon you, I suggest asking yourself these questions: "What am I afraid of? (How do I define fear in this case?) What is the worst thing that can happen? What is the best thing that can happen?" When you expose yourself long enough to face your fear, you will begin to see fear for what it really is: *powerless* without your consent and approval, and *paralyzed* without you doing all the work!

For me, fear is what happens when I lose sight of who I am and why I am here. Fear is when I retreat, rather than advance with passion. One of my past coaches once told me that fear will happen when I'm thinking about myself instead of others. Fear is a very self-centered emotion.

> *We cannot control when or how fear will come upon us, but we can control what we do with it.*

We cannot control when or how fear will come upon us, but we can control what we do with it. When fear comes upon me, I usually feel it in my stomach as a knot below my ribs. Sometimes, it disguises itself as procrastination or avoidance of something or someone. Other times, it shows up as random, revolving thoughts that cause me to lose that peaceful, easy feeling (do you know what I mean?).

When this happens, I think about what seems to be causing the fear and I move into it, instead of away from it or denying that it's there at all.

Once I recognize it, I speak to it! That's right; but not in a soft, friendly voice that invites discussion, but the way I would talk to a dog about to bite me. I command, "Go, in the name of Jesus!" Oh, how I love the name of Jesus! I can't imagine where I would be without it.

The Bible says the name of Jesus is above all other names.[1] What I hear when I read this verse is that Jesus' name is the trump card in the deck that a person has been dealt. When I was in junior high, I used to love playing the card game of Buck Euchre. We used to play it every day in the back of the bus on our way home from school. The person dealing the cards would get to bid last, and the highest bidder got to choose the trump card, which was the card that beat every other card. I loved being the highest bidder because I could look at my cards and decide which card would be the trump card.

I see God as the dealer of the cards we've been given and He says the card named Jesus is the one that beats all other cards. The best news is that we can all have access to the winning card. It trumps everything, including the card named fear! In fact (just FYI), it also conquers things like sickness, disease, obesity, sadness, poverty, discouragement, divorce, denial, depression—and the list goes on, long enough to cover everything you need. Seriously!

There are times when I will command, "Fear, get behind me!" That way, I use fear to propel me forward, instead of letting it stand in the way of where I'm going!

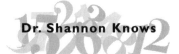

The key is, fear and faith cannot rule in the same environment. You see, fear is the opposite of faith. The way I see it is that if we operate in faith, fear has no place. This knowledge helps me rise above fear when it shows up. I remind myself that I've put my faith in a big God and I feel the power of that faith when I remember what I'm hoping for. Fear is like darkness and faith is like light; in fact, faith is light. When the light turns on, the darkness is gone!

Hopes up!

Faith is the substance of things hoped for.[2] If we keep our hopes up, we'll be able to tap into the faith that is eternally available to us. Unfortunately, most people choose to take the position of refusing to get their hopes up. We've all heard the old and far-too-popular saying, "Don't get your hopes up." Why do people say that? They say it because of fear. People are afraid of getting disappointed, hurt, let down, or not getting what they want. Once again, fear steps in the way of the one thing that has the power to ensure that our desires become reality—*hope!* Without hope, there is no faith, and without faith, fear has full authority to steal, kill, and destroy!

> ## I say, get your hopes up!
> ## You have nothing to lose except fear.

I say, get your hopes up! You have nothing to lose except fear.

I used to be very afraid of speaking in front of people. One time, I remember speaking into a microphone on stage in front of a lot of people. My heart was beating so loudly that I was absolutely sure the crowd could hear it thumping in my chest. It was horrible! That all changed once I got over what I thought people were thinking about me by focusing instead on the message I brought to share with them—a message that could save their lives!

Can you imagine what would have happened if I had allowed fear to stop me from imparting the message I was created to share? Can you imagine what would happen if you allowed fear to stop you from being who you were designed to be? It's time to expose yourself!

Knowing the truth sets us free.[3] If we want freedom, we must be willing to *know* the truth. Hope and faith are what allow us to take full authority over fear and not be held hostage by it.

A wonderful life

So, let's talk a little more about this wonderful thing called hope. Why? Because I *know* that hope is foundational to living a meaningful and fearless life of health, *wellth,* and freedom!

As a verb, *Merriam-Webster's Dictionary & Thesaurus* says "hope" is "to desire with expectation of fulfillment"; and as a noun, "hope" is "trust, reliance."[4]

What I love most about hope is the energy and momentum it creates when a person focuses on it. "Faith is being *sure* of what we hope for and *certain* of what we do not see" (italics mine).[5]

Once again, we can gain a lot of valuable insight from what this dictionary has to say about being sure and certain. "Sure" is defined as "trustworthy, reliable, and confident,"[6] while "certain" is "dependable and reliable."[7]

I'm intrigued that "sure" and "certain" are adjectives defining a person's character, and not verbs expressing a single action. Isn't it interesting that the definitions of all three words—hope, sure, and certain—have reliance/reliability in common? Therefore, all of them have to do with trustworthiness. "A reliable messenger brings healing."[8] When we become hopeful, sure, and certain in the message we share with others and ourselves, we bring healing. Hope and being sure and certain are reliable principles for health and *wellth*!

What are you sure or certain of? Have you ever asked yourself if the certainty you muster is real or a façade? If it's fake, by definition it isn't certain at all. (Again, I'm leading you to face the truth about yourself— naked and unashamed.)

Then where does that leave faith and hope?

As I said earlier, faith is the substance of that which is hoped for. The way I read and understand this is that without hope, we cannot have faith! Wow! Now that's a pretty bold statement and profound principle. If you don't know what you hope for, you cannot have faith, because faith *is* the substance or the result of what you hope for.

Hope is *not* wishful thinking. It's also not magic, although its results are beautifully magical.

Fishing, anyone?

I love to run. When I lived in Minneapolis, I would run around Lake Harriet (one of my very favorite lakes in the world) several times a week. While running early in the morning, I would always pass several men who were fishing. I would see them sitting peacefully, waiting patiently by the glassy water in anticipation of a big catch. When I would run late in the afternoon, I would see the same fishermen. They would fish there all day long!

One day I thought, "I wonder if they're catching anything?" I also wondered how long they were going to sit there on that particular day waiting for a fish to bite. Then I thought, "Imagine if they cast their lines out, but didn't use any bait. Would it change the way they sit beside Lake Harriet all day? Of course it would! Would they sit here patiently all day long? Of course they wouldn't! What makes it all worth it—the countless hours of sitting next to the water—is the anticipation of a big fish biting the bait and then reeling it in. Without the anticipation of possibility, these fishermen wouldn't sit here all day long, I'm certain of that."

Then I thought, "A healthy, *wellthy* life is kind of like fishing!"

"How?" you may ask.

What would be the difference between sitting beside a lake all day with a hook and bait in the water and catching nothing versus sitting beside the water all day simply watching the lake and obviously catching nothing? At the end of the day, the result would be the same, but the difference would be this: when you fish, you are expecting something positive! You have your hopes up.

Nobody goes fishing without expecting a bite and no one goes fishing without bait. (Although at times, with or without bait, the end result may be the same.) Even though a person is never really sure when they're going to catch a fish, no one just sits there and hopes that a fish will bite on no bait!

When you expect something, you take the necessary steps to achieve it.

So the way I see it, life is like fishing. As you go through life expecting something, you might as well expect something *big*. You might as well get your hopes up for something you'll love to remember. And I'll let you in on a little secret: You get to choose what you expect! (Big or small, good or bad.) The key component to catching a fish, or catching a great life, is hope. Know what you're fishing for and take the necessary steps to catch it—don't allow your hope to be wasted on catching something you fear.

Remember, hope means "to desire with expectation of fulfillment," so a flippant "I hope so" would be as absurd as a person fishing without bait, just sitting beside a lake and hoping to catch a fish.

What are you fishing for? What are you expecting? (What is your definition of health? What is your definition of *wellth*? What is your definition of life?) Are you using the proper bait to hook what you're trying to attract into your life?

My former pastor, Pastor Randy, used to say, "Don't pursue that which you can attract." We don't catch fish by running or swimming after them, but by taking the necessary steps to get them to come to us. Whatever you focus on, you will eventually attract into your life.

There are certain steps you need to take to increase your hope and raise your expectancy. These steps will help you immensely in your quest for knowing your *wellth* and experiencing health for life, I promise. When you *know* your *wellth*, you will prosper in health. When you *know* your *wellth*, you will transform your life. When it really comes down to it, your *wellth* is the source of your health and wealth!

Since fear is the opposite of faith and hope is necessary for faith, then what is your hope? Do you know what you hope for in your life? It's time to start dreaming. It's time to start imagining what your healthiest, best life looks like. It's time to expect a life beyond your wildest dreams! Go ahead; it's okay to desire the best that life has to offer! *No fear!*

So often when we are taught traditional goal setting, we're instructed to set a goal, and then visualize ourselves reaching that goal. Yet, it's impossible to visualize ourselves reaching that goal if we haven't been able to see, in our minds' eyes, exactly what it is we hope for.

Hope is the
foundation for successful goal achieving.

Hope is the foundation for successful goal achieving. Hope is also why the question "Is this all there is?" doesn't have to be scary at all.

So let me ask you this again, "What is it you hope for?" Because let's face it, I don't want you to set another goal and not reach it, do you? Absolutely not!

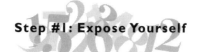

Hitting your goals

It's time to H.I.T. your goals! In my opinion, the three key components to successful goal achieving are: Hope, Inspiration, and Timing. I love acronyms, so this is an acronym I came up with years ago to turn complicated goal setting into profoundly simple goal achieving.

Goal achieving starts with *hope*. When you mix your faith with your foundation of hope, then suddenly, you have something to build on and to build with.

Please grab a pen and paper and write down specifically what it is you hope for in your life. Think about your health, your *wellth*, your family, your friendships, your work, your wealth, and whatever else it is that you hope for. (What is it you hope to experience from reading this book?) Trust me; this is going to be fun! Please don't read another word until you've done this for yourself.

Now that you've written down what you hope for, let's talk a little about *inspiration*, the second component to achieving your goals. Inspiration is the most powerfully creative force available to us. The ultimate question that inspiration answers is *why*. Why do you hope for the things you just wrote down? (What is your inspiration?) I believe your inspiration stems from who you are, and even if you're unable to eloquently write or verbalize your whys, you innately know.

Your inspiration is as natural to you as breathing. It allows life to flow as you breathe it in and live the life you are destined to live. You take a breath of inspiration, you inspire those around you, and then you ultimately expire. This is what we do as living, breathing humans! *We are designed to inspire before we expire.*

Now I want you to:

1. Take a moment to visualize your whys for what it is you hope for, and write them down.

2. Jot down all of the why nots that other, troublesome, little voices are telling you. (In Step #3, we're going to have a little meeting of the minds and settle this debate once and for all!)

The third component in achieving your goals is *timing*. Healing takes time, life takes time, and time is really nothing more than how we live. It's about time we set aside time to do what we desire to do. Yes, you read that right! If we don't make time to do what we desire to do, we won't get where we desire to go. It just won't happen!

Scheduling time to do the things you love most is essential to living a life you love and experiencing health (and *wellth*)...for life. I find it curious that most timelines have a deadline. Why do we call the date we will reach a goal a deadline? Who wants to look forward to a dreadful-sounding *dead*line? It's no wonder most people avoid setting a goal with its accompanying deadline! I am officially inviting you to join me in redefining the deadline as a *life*line and living our life on that line—the moment of mission accomplished. I say, it's about time! ☺

Lastly, I want to inform you of another definition I discovered for hope. *Merriam Webster's Dictionary* defines "HOPE" as "Health Opportunity for People Everywhere."[9] I love this (and it looks like I'm not the only one who loves acronyms)!

When you replace your fear with hope, you allow a health opportunity for people everywhere around you—including yourself.

> *"As we are liberated from our own fear,*
> *our presence automatically liberates others."*
> —*Marianne Williamson*

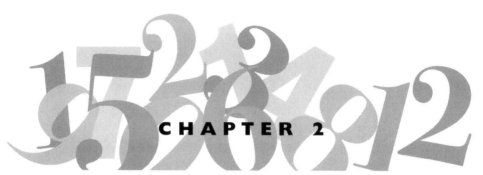

CHAPTER 2

Step #2: Locate Yourself

Did you know?

You must be willing to discover where you are, then courageous enough to embrace it.

Where are you? Now that you've taken Step #1 (Expose Yourself) and have put fear to rest, you have the power to answer this question courageously and honestly.

The most vital key for getting where you desire to go is being truthful about where you are. If you don't know where you are, it's almost impossible to get where you are going. Without knowing where you are, you may be lost and not even know it. Or you may be where you desire to be but haven't realized it yet. It's absolutely vital to know where you are on your way to where you are going!

That is what goals do for us. They define ways for us to monitor our steps as we move toward our dreams, desires, and destinations. Goals help us inspect what we expect.

If you don't know where you are, ask; but, use wisdom when asking. Who better to ask than the One with the ultimate perspective?

Where am I?

Locating yourself starts with the question (yes, the obvious question): "Where am I?" You are where you are today for a number of reasons; maybe only one or two, or the reasons may seem far too innumerable to count. One thing is for sure: I am not going to ask you why you are where you are, nor do I suggest that you do either. I have found over the years that even asking God, "Why me?" isn't very productive.

We will, however, talk about some of the reasons we step off the path that leads to a healthy, *wellthy* life. I think that we will all see that many of us have a lot more in common than we think, no matter where we are.

Sometimes, one of the most valuable insights in determining where we are stems from recognizing where we've come from.

Do the unthinkable—celebrate your successes!

Once you realize how far you've come, do the unthinkable—celebrate your successes! Doing this is so much more productive than regretting mistakes or losses.

One of my favorite chapters in the Bible is the one in the very beginning. Let's face it, this is where the original plan of the entire universe, as well as humankind, was put into motion. It absolutely fascinates me! It's also quite disturbing to discover that all of that goodness, the wonderful garden, and the daily walks with the Creator at midday were lost because of a *bad food choice*.

Okay, so maybe it wasn't necessarily just a bad food choice. Maybe it was just a bad choice, or two, or three. Let's take a look at what really happened.

The crafty serpent, which represents darkness, asked Eve a question: "Did God *really* say…?"[1] He purposely asked a question that would cause her to question what God had said, even though she knew exactly what He had said. (Could it be that where we are today, all started with a question?) This question definitely began to reveal the confusion in Eve's mind, but I don't believe it caused her confusion. You see, when God gave Adam and Eve instructions about what they could eat in the garden, He said, "You are free to eat from any tree in the garden; but you must not eat from the tree of the knowledge of good and evil, for when you eat of it, you will surely die."[2]

Just a side note here; God did not mean an instant physical death, but a spiritual death—a separation from God Himself.

What I find interesting is that when the serpent questioned Eve about what God had said, she responded with the truth. Plus a little extra. Unfortunately, she would base her decision on that extra misinformation.

The serpent then told her, "You will not surely die."[3] What he told her was true for that moment, but it wasn't the truth. According to the definition of physical death, he was correct. She would not surely die immediately after, but an important part of her would—her true self-image. This is where it gets very interesting. He told her, "For God knows that when you eat of it your eyes will be opened, and you will be like God."[4] What Eve failed to realize was that she was already like God. She was made in His very own image, which already made her like God.

Who am I?

From the very beginning, mankind has been unclear about his or her identity. I believe this has been, and still is, the basis for why we are where we are. It was this confusion that led Eve to make a decision that would not only separate her from God, but bring sin into a place that was designed to be a paradise. It was also this decision that would not only affect her life, but the lives of all humans to come.

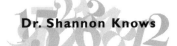

> *When we're not sure of who we are, it's easy*
> *for us to fall into wrong thinking that*
> *causes us to make bad choices.*

When we're not sure of who we are, it's easy for us to fall into wrong thinking that causes us to make bad choices. All bad choices, in my opinion, are based on confusion caused by lack of clarity. Fear interferes with clarity.

The Bible points out that "when the woman saw that the fruit of the tree was *good for food* and pleasing to the eye, and also desirable for gaining wisdom, she took some and ate it" (italics mine).[5]

Your health and *wellth*, in fact your life, depends on the food you eat. Like Eve, we all have made decisions based on what looked good for food. Food is anything that feeds us, and not always necessarily food for our stomachs. How many of us have bitten into something that looked like it would be good for food, only to find out that it was sour, bitter, or rotten? Of course, this has happened to all of us. People will make decisions based on what they believe will feed them. This is why knowing the truth about whatever it is that we are feeding on is so vital. Do not be deceived!

Eve also chose to eat the fruit because it was pleasing to the eye. This reminds me of the old sayings "beauty is only skin deep" and "not everything that glitters is gold." Or as I so often tell my daughters, "Just because it tastes good, doesn't mean it *is* good."

Eve made a bad decision because the fruit was desirable for gaining wisdom. Her desire was for wisdom, or to gain something she thought she did not have and believed she needed. What she didn't realize was that she already possessed wisdom because she had direct access to wisdom—to

God Himself—every day as she walked with Him in the garden. She also was focusing on what she thought she didn't have, instead of *knowing* and celebrating what she did!

So often we choose to do certain things because we think we will gain something or because we don't want to miss out. Let's face it, none of us wants to miss out on what we think we're entitled to. The problem is, there are a lot of counterfeits out there that are trying to copy the original or the "real deal," but they will never be able to deliver what we desire.

Lastly, Eve shared the fruit with the one closest to her. That's the problem with bad choices; eventually, they will also affect those closest to us.

Immediately, Adam and Eve no longer saw themselves as God saw them. Instead, they saw their own nakedness and were ashamed. They lost the truth and were afraid. At that point, they felt the need to cover up and hide.

Even though God knew exactly where Adam was, He called out to Adam, "Where are you?"[6] Wherever you are today, God knows exactly where you are. The key is, do you know where you are?

While visiting some friends in Houston, Texas, I wanted to get directions to a particular location, but I was the only one at the house. I couldn't even call the place I wanted to go to for directions because I knew the first thing they would ask me would be, "Where are you?" An answer of "Houston, Texas" would not be sufficient! Of course, the only way I would be able to get where I wanted to go was to first find out exactly and specifically where I was.

Locating yourself is a vital step toward getting anywhere in life, whether you are in Houston, your home, or a hospital. It's time for you to locate yourself! It's time to get honest with yourself and God about where you are. It's time for restoration, recovery, or reward. It's time to stop denying what you deserve, which is a healthy, *wellthy*, happy, abundant *you* reflected in a healthy, *wellthy*, happy, abundant life!

It isn't possible to recover, regain, retrieve, or regain normal health if you don't recognize the fact that you've lost it. In locating yourself, it is important not only to determine where you are, but where you are in relation to where you want to go.

The ultimate question is, where are you in relation to God? This is the ultimate and most critical locator. It's comforting to know that no matter where you are based on the choices you've made, you are just one decision and one step away from finding or returning to Him. In fact, He may be calling out to you right now, "Where are you?"

It is essential for you to ask yourself, "Where am I, and how do I see myself?" The answers will lead you to your next step.

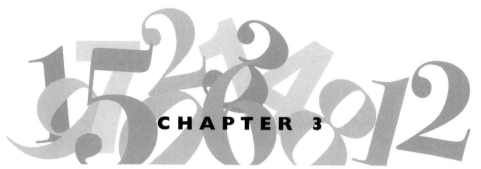

CHAPTER 3

Step #3: Know Yourself

Did you know?

*If you delight in the Lord,
He will give you the desires of your heart.*[1]

What do you desire?

Knowing what you desire is essential for living a life of health and *wellth*. You must know yourself and K.N.O.W. (Know Now Or Want) for yourself. In other words, know what you desire now or continue to live in a state of want. Seriously, this is usually where most people will shrink back, stop or stay, and not move ahead. Your best time is *now*! If this step makes you nervous, then you are not alone, but if it makes you scared (you are still not alone), go back to Step #1 and Expose Yourself once again. Be encouraged, *you* can know exactly what it is you desire. You have permission to admit what it is you desire and you have what it takes to receive it.

It's true. In order to get to where you are going, it is vital to know where you are right now. Then you must define where you are going. Where are you going? Where do you desire to go? What are the desires of your heart?

The majority of the time I ask people what they desire, they quickly respond, "I don't know." With all due respect, I do not believe this is true. If you are one of these people, I encourage you to contemplate this. You *do know*! It's just a matter of your desires rising to a conscious level or becoming courageous enough to acknowledge what you innately know. I like to refer to it as "the knowing."

> ### Knowing what you desire doesn't mean you have to know how it's going to happen.

May I share a little something with you that changed my life years ago and has continued to influence me numerous times since then? Knowing what you desire doesn't mean you have to know how it's going to happen. (It doesn't? Nope, it doesn't!) In fact, the more I dare to know and freely declare my desires, the clearer the how-tos become.

A major thing I have discovered in my life is the power of perspective. Sometimes just one little distinction causes a vital shift in my perspective that radically transforms my thinking. My hope is that this is already happening for you and will continue to, especially in this step.

When I discovered the distinct difference between a want and a desire, I gained a valuable new perspective. *Merriam-Webster's Dictionary & Thesaurus* defines the verb "want" as: "1. to fail to possess: LACK 2. to feel or suffer the need of 3. NEED, REQUIRE, WISH. As a noun, "want" is 1. a lack of a required or usual amount: SHORTAGE 2. dire need: DESTITUTION 3. something wanted 4. personal defect: FAULT."[2]

The verb "desire" is defined as: "1. to long or hope for: exhibit or feel desire for 2. REQUEST."[3] The word "desire" comes from the Latin word *desiderare*, which means "heavenly body."[4] (How cool is that?)

Do you notice the difference between these two words? Even though we use these words interchangeably all the time, "want" seems to be so negative, so "not enough," so "wanting." Desire, on the other hand, is much more positive. A heavenly body—enough said!

Long story short, you must know what you desire. Know now or be in a state of want. Quite simply, KNOW!

Mission possible

For this step, I am going to take you back to a revelation I had on October 14, 2007, that radically transformed my thinking. It helped me embrace what I know, and the critical difference between knowing and wanting. Before I share it with you, I want to remind you that I personally believe that deep down everyone *knows* what it is they truly desire. It's there! It has been there since the beginning of time. I also believe that God gives us the desires of our hearts. That's one of the reasons I believe that these desires have been there since the beginning of time. Before we were formed in our mothers' wombs, God knew us.[5] He knew who we were then, and He knows who we are now! He put desires in our "who" and then commissioned us to "do." He gave us each a mission, then designed us wonderfully and magnificently to accomplish that mission. The knowing is there because the *all-knowing* One put it there. The gifts and abilities we need to accomplish this mission are already present and available to us from within us.

What are you willing to be, do, and have in your life?

Once you're ready, this next step is part of the process of preparing yourself for the fullest expression of your God-given possibilities, where your hopes, dreams, and desires become a reality—your healthy, *wellthy* life. As you are willing and ready to express them, you will get what you desire. The key here is willingness. What are you willing to be, do, and have in your life? Are you willing and ready to live the life you desire? That, my friend, is the zillion-dollar question!

This is where fear stops most people from answering. So often, we're afraid to admit our deepest desires because we think we won't get what we want (or I should say, "desire"), or we think that once we proclaim our desires, somehow it's up to us to figure out all the intricate details and make them happen. Now, that's not only scary, but stressful—am I right? (I believe I am!) That's one reason we've done Step #1 (Expose Yourself), and we will continue to do Step #1 as often as fear rears its ugly head.

Often, we get so caught up in trying to figure out the how-tos that we never get quiet long enough to allow the known desires from deep within us to speak. When this happens, we either stand motionless—paralyzed by our fear, confusion, and indecision—or we frantically run in circles, only to vainly chase a wind that eludes us.

"The knowing" is where it gets quite profound, if you let it. Knowing has very little to do with your head and everything to do with your heart. In fact, knowing is when your head finally connects with your heart, where the you on the inside is reflected in the you on the outside. The ultimate way to acknowledge the knowing is by acknowledging the One who knows. Seriously, in order to answer the calling in your life, or to fulfill the purpose you have for being on this wonderful planet, knowing the One who knows is absolutely essential! It is why I am even here today and it's why I am able to share my purpose with you. I believe I've been specifically designed to share this message of hope with you today.

The Bible says "perfect love drives out fear."[6] This is the ultimate answer to eradicating fear in your life. Put perfect love *all* over it. Keep reading...this is going to make perfect sense, I promise! You see, your purpose and your desires are not just for you. Will they bless you? Absolutely—beyond your wildest dreams; but that is because you are blessed to be a blessing. If you don't fulfill the purpose in your life and receive the true desires of your heart, everyone loses, including you.

You have greater influence on this planet than you realize. Who is going to benefit from your knowing and getting what you desire? Who is going to benefit from your fulfillment of your God-given destiny and purpose? All of us! Whether you like to admit it or not, knowing what you desire is absolutely vital.

Let me ask another way. Who is going to miss out because you haven't yet discovered or acknowledged your knowing? Who is going to miss out if you don't get what you desire? Who is going to suffer if you don't fulfill your God-given destiny and purpose? We all are, especially you and those closest to you.

So let's take a step back in time to October 14, 2007. I will show you what I learned that has helped me immensely in this step of knowing what I desire, and ultimately getting it:

October 14, 2007, journal entry

This morning while praying, I was thinking about and talking to God about why I have been so angry lately, and asking God to help me with this. I realized that two things seem to make me angry:

1) When I don't feel loved or respected; and, 2) When I don't get what I want. This is not always the situation, but sometimes. Then, it came to me…a limiting belief that I have: I need to get what I want to be happy. (Who says so? Where did this come from? Is it true? I guess it has been.)

What God showed me is the difference between getting what I want and knowing what I desire. WOW! Knowing what I desire will come from truly loving myself enough to admit to myself what it is that I truly desire, and truly allowing myself to know it because I know me and the

God who created me. Then when I truly know what I desire, I won't get so angry when I don't get what I want, because I know and trust that I will get what I desire when I am ready. When I know what I desire, I will be able to "receive and embrace" it when it does come. You see, if I don't know what I desire, I will either not recognize it when it does show up or it will totally scare me because it is not something I know. Therefore, it is an unknown, and naturally, the unknown feels unfamiliar and scary. This is why it is so important to know and to allow myself to know, so that I am able to receive it, experience it, and celebrate it when I do get it.

How do I do that? By first loving myself enough to embrace my desires and get to know them. How? By allowing myself to know Shannon with no judgment; to love her as is. When I do this, I will be able to love others more deeply also, as is. If I can love myself as is, then I don't necessarily have to get what I want to be happy. What do I mean by this? I will love her regardless of whether she does what I want her to do moment by moment, minute by minute; regardless of whether or not she gives me exactly what I want, or her life gives me exactly what I want right now. Instead, I love her just because she's loveable.

(I do desire to love myself enough to truly know myself, genuinely, consciously, deeply. WOW!! Lord, show me those areas that I do not love about myself and either remove them from me or allow me to love them...in the now, please!)

So, my new belief is: 'I need to know what I desire to be happy. I need to love myself, to know what I truly desire. I need to know and love God to truly love and know myself. So when I know God, I can love God, and when I love Him, I can love Shannon; and when I love Shannon, I can KNOW her. When I love others, then others will love me. It's that simple! It really is true that we must first love ourselves in order to truly love others.

Instead, I have been making the love I have for me dependent on only what I know of me, but if judgment and fear have gotten in the way of *me truly knowing me, I haven't been able to love me. But now I see, thanks to God's light of revelation, that when I love me, then I will be able to know me, because perfect love casts out all fear…and when I know, I will get what I desire…the truth. That is, the truth about me and my life; which is that I am more than enough, and that I am abundant. I am free to be truly me! I live in freedom and prosperity, the goodness and fullness of God Almighty.*

(Praise God!! Thank you so much, my dear and loving God; you are the best!!! I love you with all of me. Help me to love me with all of you. I don't need to get what I want to be happy. I AM HAPPY! When I can get beyond a feeling, this is where I will get my healing! Beyond the feeling is the healing. I have been afraid to be specific. Most people are.)

This is why most have never yet gotten what they truly desire. This is why so many people never reach goals because they are merely needs or wants and not specific. Until it is specific, it is merely a want or a wish. This is also why people are afraid to set goals because it makes them be specific, and with fear, they cannot be.

This has been so true in my own life. When I need to get what I want to be happy, I will not be; nor will I get what I truly desire. I do not need to get what I desire to be happy. When I know what I desire, not only am I happy, but also eventually I get what I desire. When I know what I desire, I don't NEED to get it, but I do.

I have seen this in my own life so many times. When I KNOW, I get. When I want, I don't. When I want, I just end up wanting more. With regards to being specific, based on my past limiting beliefs, I have been afraid to be specific because I had not been getting what I desire, but now I see that this is exactly why; it's from not being specific. Why? It's because of the fear that my past limiting belief has caused me to have. Wow! When I don't know what I desire (consciously) and love myself enough to admit it, I will not get it. This is the key. The key is KNOWING specifically.

People will say that they do not know what they desire, but everyone knows unconsciously. It is not until we love ourselves enough to know that we will KNOW.

The Board Meeting

There is a powerful difference between needing and knowing. You need because you do not know, but when you know, you do not need. What is God calling you to *know* right now? If the answer is anything but specific and positive, my question to you is, who told you that? Seriously, *"Who told you that?"*

A dear friend of mine told me about an experience he had that resulted in helping him conquer financial lack. He then shared it with me (thanks, Brant) and now I'm going to pass it on to you. This experience changed my life, and it will do the same for you if you let it. Do not, I repeat, do not go on to the next step without doing this exercise. Allow yourself to fully experience it. Once you do, take the time necessary to write down your experience, just like I did. It will not only help you, but those you share it with. I promise! By the way, the day after I had this experience that I call "The Board Meeting," I saw the friend who originally told me about it. He said that when I walked into the room, he could instantly see a difference in me. He said I looked like I almost glowed; I looked so light and free! My hope is that you will as well. Enjoy your meeting! (When you finish, I have included my experience for you to enjoy, and perhaps it will bless you, too.)

What I want you to do is envision a boardroom. I want you to just get a feel for what the room is like, what the table is like, how many chairs there are, where the doors are, where the windows are, if any. What color are the walls? The table?

Next, I want you to slowly invite the people into the room who have made you feel "less than"—unworthy, afraid, and insecure. By making this open invitation, you are inviting individuals you may not be consciously aware of to come and join you. You may be somewhat surprised when they show up.

As they come in, allow them to sit down at the boardroom table. One by one, they will come. Welcome them in. They may be past friends; they may be the people closest to you. They may be coworkers, relatives, or maybe even a kindergarten teacher. Whoever they are, welcome them into the room. Welcome them into your boardroom.

Now what I want you to do is this: I want you to take a moment, and go to each person individually. I want you to let them know how their words affected you. I want you to let them know how their actions have affected you. I want you to be present with each person in the moment, until you get to the point where you feel like you've said all that you need to say, felt all that you need to feel, and you are ready to forgive and release them.

Forgiveness will prepare you for your next step of health (and *wellth)* for life. You can do it! I promise. I believe that as long as you hold unforgiveness in your heart toward anyone, including yourself, you will be unable to know exactly what it is that you truly desire. Unforgiveness will get in the way of really loving and knowing your true self, and it will also cause a lot of unnecessary fear!

When you forgive a person, move to the next one. One by one, I want you to have a conversation with every person in the room, and when you are finished, I want you to very graciously dismiss everybody from the room and thank them for coming. Release them to go on with their lives, and now release yourself to go forward with yours.

Do yourself a favor; set down this book, close your eyes, and fully experience what I'm talking about. As soon as you are finished, write down all the details about what you've experienced and what you've learned. (If you would like for me to help you by guiding you through this visualization, go to www.drshannonknows.com.)

This is my story of my board meeting, but please do not read this until you have had your own meeting (I do not want my experience to influence or limit your personal experience in any way, *please*!):

This morning I gathered together everyone who has ever helped me feel insecure, less than, or not good enough.

We met in a pale yellow conference room with a large brown table. At first it seemed as though there were not going to be very many people in attendance. But as people continued to come, everyone had to shift to their right and make room. By the time we were finished, there were no more seats at the table—it was full!

I went around the room and, one by one, I told them how I felt or what I thought. I forgave them or asked them to forgive me. Some of them I really felt almost sorry for…I felt compassion for who they were and the hurts that they too had experienced in their own lives. As soon as there was peace between us, I moved to the next person. I felt love toward everyone in that room, even those who had really hurt me!

The last person to walk through the door was Shannon, and did she look good! She was radiant! She looked so happy. She was glowing, and her presence was so big and inviting! Wow, what an amazing transformation! She was smiling so beautifully and her lips glistened with a glossy shine. Her eyes sparkled. Her hair was long, straight, and very blonde. Her hair looked so shiny and healthy. It flowed away from her head as she swiftly entered the room. Her arms were out to the side, as if to welcome me, as well as to invite a hug at the same time. She was so glad to be seen and very glad to also see me!

We hugged for a long time. We told each other how much we loved each other. I apologized for not fully recognizing her in my life. She apologized for not fully expressing herself! We forgave each other and I told her how wonderful it was to see her. I also told her how beautiful, fascinating, and more than enough she was. She thanked me and said that I was free to go! But before I left, I made a broad statement to everyone else who may be outside of those doors, "It's OK, you are all free to go!"

Everyone else peacefully followed me out of the room. Shannon (the new Shannon who is beautiful and free) stayed in the room…so happy, so grateful! The room was glowing. God, Jesus, and the Holy Spirit were all there sitting at the head of the table where I (the old Shannon who was not enough) had once sat. They told her that they were proud of her. She smiled and asked that if anyone else came into the room, perhaps someone whom she had forgotten to invite, to please let them know that they too were released and were free to go.

Before she (now ME…the beautiful new Shannon who is free, fascinating, and more than enough!) left, they assigned six angels to go with me to minister and help me…to walk with me in my life. The angel of beauty came upon me and entered my being from my head, down. To my left is wisdom, and to my right is insight. Behind me is discernment to guard my back, and the angel of love is in front of me. "But where is understanding?" I asked. "I need understanding." I was told that she would go before me, and around me…wherever she was needed at the time. As I walked out that door, I was surrounded with a cloud of peace. As the door shut behind me, I saw a glow of light coming from under the door. I do not think I will need to return to that room, but if I do, I know who will be there to help me.

This experience was the beginning of my journey toward living the truth, because it helped me *know* the truth. I hope it does the same for you, too.

May I share another little secret with you? You can do a board meeting at any time and for any reason—whether it's sickness, sadness, or suffering. For example, if you have been suffering with financial lack or poverty thinking, find out why. Ask yourself, "Who in my life has told me things or done things to me that caused me to feel invaluable? Unsuccessful? Sick? Fearful? Poor? That money is the root of all evil?"

Did you know that money is not evil or the root of all evil? Instead, it's the *love* of money that is! There is a big difference.

There is a distinct difference between what we "think" we know and what we truly know *deep in our hearts*. Sometimes, what you think you know is not the truth. That difference can create a conflict that causes so much inside interference that you no longer know what you desire, what you know, or what you think anymore. Sometimes, you may be absolutely convinced that what you know about yourself or others is the truth when it is not.

The longer you believe a lie, the more real it will become to you, because what you believe will be reflected in your life. Unconsciously, you will be looking for evidence that supports the lie, and you may actually begin to build a pretty believable case for yourself…or I should say, against yourself. Sadly, you will become more convinced that you are the one who is not enough, and the idea of living an abundant, healthy, *wellthy* life will seem like an impossibility.

Of everything you believe, ask yourself, "Who said that?"

Of everything you believe, ask yourself, "Who said that?" Especially when it's a belief that seems to be limiting your possibilities or choices. One day when I was sharing this with my mentor, he said, "I love that question. I always tell people to ask, 'Who said it?' of everything they believe. Then they will know whether or not to believe it." (Thanks, John

Mason!) Guess what, *you* get to decide what you are going to believe. And your beliefs will not only create your destination, but they will be the way you get there; your beliefs act not only as your road map, but as the vehicle and the gas that will be required to get you to your destination.

How many of us have gone through life thinking that what we believe is truth, and we think we know, when in fact, we may not? I encourage you right now to think about what you "think" you know; what you believe. Then ask yourself, "Who told me that?" Invite those people to join you in your boardroom. Perhaps it's time to let some things go or let someone go! Just look at them lovingly and say, "You're fired! It's not personal, it's just business—my business." ☺

Perhaps it's time for you to trade in your busyness for the business that God sent you here to attend to.

Restful restoration

Years ago, I felt like God was trying desperately to get me the message: Rest Shannon, rest. Being a very busy, active person, I was very bothered by this message. In fact, looking back, it seemed to be the beginning of one of the busiest times of my life. It seemed as the though the more I tried to be obedient and rest, the more restless and busy I became. Frankly, I was so bothered by it all that I began to get frustrated. I just didn't know exactly how to rest! Needless to say, the more frustrated I became, the more restless and busy my life became and I became extremely exhausted, inside and out. I was running at warp speed and I didn't know how to stop or even slow down. The more I tried to rest, the further behind I seemed to get, which caused me to become even more restless.

My life and my schedule seemed to be spinning out of control. I was so tired; mentally, emotionally, and physically. My questions, "How did this happen, and what can I do about it?" fed my frustration and restlessness even more. It seemed as though I didn't have enough time, money, joy, or rest. And I just couldn't comprehend how lying around all day resting on the couch (eating bonbons ☺) was going to help matters, although I did try a couple times (minus the bonbons). Come to think of it, I did eat things I wouldn't normally eat while I was sitting on that couch and they didn't seem to help at all!

When we dare to KNOW, that is where we find rest.

I was determined to get the answer to the burning question on the inside of me, "What do you mean by rest, God?" After traveling halfway around the world (how's that for resting?), I finally got the answer I was looking for. When I told one of my mentors about this message that I had been getting from God, but was so unsure of the answer, he responded so simply, "Oh, that's easy. Rest means getting into agreement with God." It was one of the biggest aha moments of my life. I finally got it! It made total sense to me. Come to realize it, traveling halfway around the world was actually one of the most restful things I had done up until that point because it had been a desire of mine for a long time. And it was this desire that led me to get into agreement with God and finally get the rest I so desperately needed. Perhaps it was why I discovered the answer to the question that seemed to be driving me that instead turned out to be leading me to the truth. When we dare to KNOW (know our desires and live them), that is where we find rest.

In order to get into agreement with God, you must get into agreement with the truth that is inside of you; the truth about you! If you do not know that truth, or haven't acknowledged the truth because you've been afraid to (go back to Step #1), it will be impossible to agree. And the result will be frustrated restlessness.

The greatest news is this: It is possible to know the truth, and it is this knowing that will set you free!

Do nothing

A patient of mine (let's refer to him as Mr. Woods) was complaining of a strange feeling in his head that felt like a heavy fogginess that seemed to almost be overtaking him. I asked him if he would describe it as a headache. He cautiously answered by saying, "No, but…" It was the "but" that I found so interesting.

He told me how this feeling in his head reminded him of something that happened to him several years ago. For twenty-two months, he suffered from a severe headache. Nothing seemed to give him relief. He saw several different professionals, none of which seemed to have the answer. They prescribed numerous drugs that not only did not help, but made matters worse. With all the comprehensive testing that he went through, the overwhelming result was that no one could tell him the cause of his twenty-two months of unstoppable pain. It seemed as though there was no medically known cause for his problem. Off the record, his diagnosis was, "It's all in your head." He already knew that!

But what he didn't know was that all he needed to do was nothing. After being referred for counseling, his counselor said that the prescription for his condition was to do nothing, literally. The counselor explained that his brain had become so overloaded that it was like a computer that was in desperate need of a rebooting. He was sent to Florida for a week to intentionally do nothing. What? This sounds like a great *Seinfeld* episode, doesn't it?

When I asked him about his week in Florida, he said that he sat by a pond and just looked at it for the entire week. He did not play golf, read, or anything else that people would define as "relaxing." He literally did nothing.

Did it help? Absolutely! He said that shortly after doing nothing, the twenty-two-month headache began to leave his head. For months afterward, he maintained his balance with regular and relaxing golf outings and moments of intentionally doing nothing.

"If you don't currently have a headache, how did that experience resemble the fogginess you're currently experiencing?" I asked.

He quickly responded, "It just reminds me of the feeling I had at that time."

"What feeling?" I asked.

"The overwhelming feeling of not being able to explain why my head feels the way it does, and not being able to get rid of it," he replied, almost hopelessly.

Then I asked what seemed to be the obvious, "So, have you been practicing the art of doing 'nothing' on a regular basis?"

His reply was a convicted, "Of course not!"

You'll never guess what I told him to do (yeah, right)! I told him that he needs to do a little more nothing, and if need be, a whole lot of nothing. He agreed. After only a couple golf outings and some intentional nothingness, which allowed his head to get quiet and still, he said that he noticed a considerable improvement in the fog that had been plaguing him for several months.

Can it really be that simple? Yes, it can. Once you *know* the truth, you can rest and you can move ahead in that rest boldly and beautifully, with momentous action. That's when you will see how rest is the biggest part of restoration.

I am so excited for you and what is about to happen for you. Trust me, it is so worth the journey of many steps!

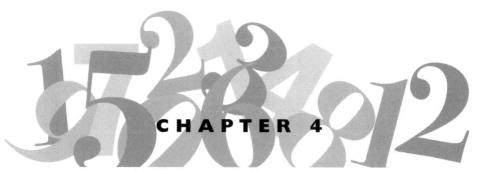

CHAPTER 4

Step #4: Be Answerable

Did you know?

When you take responsibility for your failures, you can also be responsible for your success.

Responsibility. Who likes this word besides parents, preachers, and teachers?

No one, unless they learn the true meaning of the word! According to the dictionary, "responsibility" is: 1. liable to be called upon to answer for one's acts or decisions: ANSWERABLE 2. RELIABLE, TRUSTWORTHY.[1]

Notice those words "reliable" and "trustworthy" coming up again. That's interesting, isn't it? I had no idea that being responsible is the same as being sure and certain. That is great! I'm going to summarize by saying that by simply taking our responsibility, we are becoming sure and certain (see Step #1 Expose Yourself). When we mix this with hope, the result is faith. And guess what? Faith has the power to move mountains. Do you have any mountains in your life that need moving? Perhaps *you* may be one of those mountains.

Did you know that wherever you are today, whatever circumstance or situation you're in, somewhere along the way, you chose it? ("What, are you kidding me?" you say.)

When someone told me this years ago, I was shocked, and quite honestly, I was mad. "How dare anyone tell me that I'm responsible for the situation I'm in?" I thought. The truth was, once I began to look at the past "conclusions" or so-called "truths" that I had accepted in my heart as true, my role in the circumstances that I was dealing with made a lot more sense.

A lot of times when we are in a very painful, emotional situation, we will choose a certain way of thinking to protect ourselves, our egos, or our feelings (again, what are you certain about?). The problem is, if we're not thinking the truth, that so-called "protection" will someday become our prison.

When you resign yourself to a conclusion that takes away your choices, free will, or ability to respond, you become powerless. And when the power goes out, your light extinguishes and so do you! Blame is definitely a conclusion that serves no one, especially not you.

You are probably wondering what the word "serve" actually means. I did too. Check this definition out: "to furnish or supply with something (one power company serving the whole state)."[2] (I'm not kidding, that's what the dictionary says.) It's awesome.

You see, our conclusions are either serving those around us and ourselves, or they are not. We get to choose.

Your truth will become your reality...period. But what if you have believed something that is simply not true? Well, I've got good news for you; it doesn't have to stay that way!

Do not come to a conclusion that doesn't serve you. At first glance, that may seem a little selfish or self-centered. However, if you look deeper, as I had to, you will see that deeper doesn't mean more complex. Quite to the contrary, everything becomes simpler. Basic truths or "principles," as I like to call them, are fundamental and foundational. They allow us to stand firmly rooted in something that serves us *and* the greater good. If you don't stand for something, you'll fall for anything. If you do not stand firmly on something, you will fall, at *any time* and eventually, *every time*.

Responsibility means "using our ability to respond." Now, I must give credit where credit is due: I heard someone say something similar to this before, so I'm not taking the credit for it. In fact, the exact thing I heard was "the ability to respond," although I'm not sure where I heard this. However, I think using our ability to respond is somewhat of an original idea. Nonetheless, whether I came up with it or not, it's good. Don't you think? ☺

> ### When we own our own mistakes,
> ### we can own our own successes.

Once you recognize your abilities and the power that lies within you, you can respond. And when you do respond with your ability, the massive actions that can take place will absolutely catapult you into the life of your dreams! So often when we take a look at our lives and we are unhappy with what we see, the natural tendency is to blame someone, especially someone other than ourselves (or we beat up on ourselves). This is exactly *not* what taking responsibility is all about. When we own our own mistakes, we can own our own successes. As long as we put someone else in charge of our failure, we put someone else in charge of our success.

Your success or lack of it, your happiness or lack of it, your health or lack of it, your *wellth* or lack of it *is not* someone else's responsibility; it is yours!

I encourage you right now to take a mental inventory of your life. See it for what it really is, especially now that you have exposed your fears, located yourself, and admitted your desires. You know what you desire, so is there any area of your life where there is lack in any form? A lack of peace, health, *wellth*, happiness, joy, wealth—whatever you desire, honestly identify it now.

Think about it. Get quiet and ask yourself, "Is this what I desire?" Ask yourself, "Is this something I am responsible for?"

Stop right there. Did that last question make you mad or offended? Great! Then I can assure you, there is healing and breakthrough on the other side of your offense, and if you take responsibility now, you can move through it. Remember, "breakthrough" is all about "going through." Are you ready to go through to your breakthrough? You can do it!

Of course, if something bad happened to you as a child, very likely you are not responsible for any of it. (And if you've been carrying around the shame of blaming yourself, it is time to let yourself go free!) Sometimes we aren't responsible for what happened, *but* we are definitely responsible for what happens next.

The victim mentality will do more harm to your life than any other. You are not a victim! No matter what has happened to you, or is happening to you, you can be victorious!

No victim here

Not long ago, I was listed on a police report as a "victim." When I saw the report and my name on the line that said, "Name of Victim," it bothered me so much that I felt almost as bad about it as I did about the crime itself. I just could not get it out of my head.

A couple days later, my daughter, Anni, and I were discussing what had happened, and I was encouraging her to look at the whole situation from a point of victory and empowerment versus being a victim. She totally agreed. Then suddenly at the same time, we both commented about how it felt to see my name listed as a victim on the police report. She told me that when she saw it, she thought, "Oh boy, I bet my mom didn't like being called a victim!" Then she said, "Mom, I saw that and I was thinking, 'What? My mom's not a victim. No one died here. There's no victim. My mom's not a victim!'" I was so moved to hear her perspective. But what inspired me most were her comments, "No one died here. There is no victim."

Do you realize that when you give yourself over to being the victim, something dies? That's right, a piece of you dies—the ability to take responsibility for your situation and the accompanying power to move past your loss into victory and gain.

Responsibility is the key to your restoration.

What got you to where you are today? I tell people that "getting well is like getting un-well in reverse." Responsibility is the key to your restoration. Rest, get quiet, and see yourself where you are, because you are where you are! (Or as I like to say, "It is what it is!") You cannot undo the past, but you can do your today and your future by allowing your abilities to respond to where you are today and where you desire to be tomorrow. Now is all you have.

Stop making excuses, stop feeling sorry for yourself, and make the most of what you have right here, right now!

Please know that even though this sounds tough, it is the truth. As far as I am concerned, the most helpful and loving thing I can do for you is to tell you the truth. Remember, a reliable messenger brings healing.[3]

Before I say one more thing, I need to tell you something because I don't want you to misunderstand me. I also believe there is a time for tears; there is a time to feel the pain and there is a time to allow feelings of hurt. It is absolutely vital that you press into the pain and not push it away or run from it. I tell my patients all the time, "You got to feel it to heal it." This is exactly the opposite of what everybody else tells us, especially when it comes to pain. Pain is a sign that you are alive and once you embrace it, I promise it won't feel so bad.

Sometimes a good cry is all you need. Yes, you too, Mr. Macho Man. Then it's time to do what I tell myself to do, "Put your big girl (or big boy) pants on and deal with it!"

Make a decision right now that you are going to make right the wrongs that are within your power. For those things that are not in your power to make right, let God make them right for you, with His power. Let go of those who have wronged you, and make a right decision today to move beyond the wrongs of the past. Base this decision on where you see yourself today, keeping in mind tomorrow, or next year, or the next ten years. After going through Steps #1-#3, you are now fearless (or at least aware of your fears) and know what you desire. You know where you are and where you're going.

What must you do today, right now, to take the next step toward the future you desire? This is your game plan for success.

Taking responsibility allows for massive action. You finally have the power and permission to take authority over your life and take powerful, productive action. You can see exactly what you desire your results to be, and clearly see the steps that take you there, which is a much easier and a lot more fun way to live than adopting a victim mentality.

Traditional success teaching will tell us that we have to visualize what we want. In my experience, it has been very difficult to do that without first facing my fears, identifying where I am, admitting where I desire to go, and above all, taking responsibility for where I am and where I'm going. Unless you take these steps first, you won't be able to see what you are trying to visualize (if you can't see it, you can't visualize it). Instead, you will continue to unsuccessfully "try" to visualize what you "want," which just creates more "want." When you begin to allow yourself to see the desires you hold deep in your heart, the vision for your life will become so crystal clear that seeing (visualizing) it will be almost effortless.

When you're taking the necessary steps to live a healthy, *wellthy* life, visualizing is an important and natural part of it. What you desire for your life is what you must visualize. And when you see it, your "vision" will be clear, your steps will become very clear, and your vision will become your reality.

Seeing your desires

For the last several years, with the help of a phenomenal team, I, along with a group of dedicated volunteers, have put on a major community event. That first year, in order to be prepared for and execute the event, I had to *see* it happening from beginning to end. I set a timeline and walked through every detail of it. For example, I visualized walking into the building and I saw that we needed greeters at the door to welcome our guests. Therefore, Action #1 was "get greeters." Then, I visualized them sitting at a table, so Action #2 was "make sure we have two chairs and a table at the front door for the greeters." Then I thought, "How will people know they are at the right event?" That resulted in Action #3: "make a sign that says '*health4life REVOLUTION!* TRANSFORMATION CHALLENGE.' Each time I saw something we needed, I set another action in place in order to execute our event. Do you see what I mean?

Earlier, when I asked you what exactly you desire and why you desire it, you may have had difficulty answering this (but by now you're getting better at it, right?). It's all about your perception: What are you willing to see? What are you willing to respond to?

Since taking responsibility is about taking massive action, you may be saying to yourself, "But I don't know how," to which I say, "Yes, you do!" Do you know how I know this? Because I'm absolutely sure you've been on a vacation, planned a weekend getaway, and followed a recipe, or at least desired to be on a vacation and to make a batch of old-fashioned cookies.

How hard was it to desire a dream vacation? How hard was it to see what you would need to do to make it happen? How hard was it to experience it happening in your mind's eye? It was hard only if you lost sight of the goal or started making excuses about why it couldn't happen and started blaming others.

Face it, once you've ever made up your mind that something was going to happen no matter what, all of the details just seemed to come to mind and make sense, and it eventually happened, right?

Simply taking the next best step will get you there.

Even if you don't know all the steps to make something occur, simply taking the next best step will get you there, if you're clear about where you're going and you stay headed in that direction. Have you ever noticed how much you can accomplish the day or week before you leave on vacation? That is what I'm talking about!

Stop making excuses. Stop blaming. Stop pointing fingers and start dreaming, planning, and preparing for great things to happen—*please!* My coach and mentor, Dr. Schiffman, tells me, "Excuses are like toilets. We all have them and they all stink." Yes, we all have reasons for why this has happened or that hasn't happened, blah, blah, blah. Maybe this seems like a whole new concept. So how about joining me in this new way of living?

Taking a step

This way of living reminds me of one of my patients whom I will call Mac. I met Mac at Women's Health Expo, of all places. He hobbled up to me with his right leg in a walking cast, he was bald, at least one hundred pounds overweight, and about six foot five. He was huge! He had a lot of questions and concerns regarding his health, with good reason.

After checking his nervous system for interference caused by *vertebral subluxation* (spinal misalignment), I recommended that he come in to my office for a thorough spinal examination and X-rays. He agreed, but only after asking if my office was open on Saturdays and making it very clear to me that he had no job, no money, and went to school five days a week from morning until night. I told him that I was normally not open on Saturdays, but would be happy to see him the following Saturday at my office. I told him not to worry about the details, but to start with one step and we would determine the next best step from there. He agreed.

After evaluating him in my office, I found numerous spinal misalignments that were causing significant nerve interference. I also discovered that he was diabetic, had a horribly unhealthful diet, and was not exercising at all. His broken ankle was the least of his worries!

Even though we weren't typically open on Saturdays and he had no job and no money, he found a way to not only come to the office to be adjusted several times a week, but to pay for an entire year of care! *Mac found a way once he stopped looking at what he couldn't do and started doing what he could do.*

He made incredible improvements in his health, including losing thirty pounds in ninety days by applying the steps I am sharing with you. He transformed from the inside out by making adjustments to the way he was living. He began exercising, even though he had a broken ankle. (Yes, that's right.) I told him that even though his ankle didn't work, his arms did; so I ordered him an inexpensive tabletop bike and he pedaled it with his arms. He moved what he could, and it moved him to a level of health he had never experienced before.

Several months after he began care in my office, he was scheduled for his third and final ankle reconstruction surgery. His body (and mind) were functioning so optimally that his doctor released him from the hospital early and said that he had never seen anyone heal so quickly. In fact, Mac told me that when his doctor took off his bandages the day after surgery, his only two words were "Holy ****" because he could not believe that there was no swelling in Mac's ankle or leg! We laughed because we knew that he had witnessed holy healing and it was because Mac was finally caring for his body the way God intended. There was no more mention of "possible amputation" from his doctor.

Although Mac had a lot of reasons not to exercise, including a broken ankle, he got his body moving. Although he had a lot of reasons not to follow through with the chiropractic care that I recommended, including no time, no money, and no job, he followed through and never missed a single visit in over a year! He took responsibility for his health and has experienced great health and *wellth* ever since.

Several months into his care I invited him to be a guest speaker at a special workshop I was hosting for our annual *health4life REVOLUTION!* TRANSFORMATION CHALLENGE participants. Because it's a twelve-week community fitness challenge, the participants were referring to it as only a twelve-week program, yet they were doing the same program that Mac was doing. When he got up to share his personal story about how the "health4life" program had changed his life, he looked around very seriously and said, "I didn't realize that this was a twelve-week program. I thought this was for a lifetime, because I knew that this was about not only living my best life, but also saving it. And why would anyone want to live their best life for only twelve weeks?"

For a lifetime

What you hold in your hands is not just a twelve-week program, but twelve powerful steps that will radically transform your life and help you "get with the program." These twelve steps will become a way of living that starts with a reprogramming of your current "program" or a redirecting of your current steps, and will help you walk out the life you were born to live (if you are willing).

What I have found is that if you do Steps #1-#3 (Expose Yourself, Locate Yourself, Know Yourself), and then take responsibility, life gets so much easier. Please take a moment and make some decisions right now. What are you willing to do to get what you know you desire? Are you willing to leave the past behind? Are you willing to forgive others? Are you willing to forgive yourself? (*This is vastly important!*) Are you willing to stop being a victim? Are you willing to be victorious? Are you willing to commit to being the best you that you can be? Ask yourself, "What am I willing to do today? What am I willing to do in tomorrow's today?" Don't worry, the step-by-step part is coming, but unless you do this step, the rest doesn't matter.

Take a moment to reflect on these questions, and then grab a piece of paper and answer them. *If you're at all like me, you're probably saying, "But just tell me what to do and I will do it. Where is the plan?"* Please listen to me. You are beginning to write it, right now. Health for life is not just another program, diet, or plan. It is *your* life. It is *your* purpose. It is *your* plan! This is the plan for your life! It's about health and *wellth* for a lifetime, in all areas of your life.

The absence of pain or feeling well is not health or wellth!

Health does not come from the outside in, even though this is what we are told every time we open a magazine, newspaper, or turn on the television or radio. We are programmed every day by drug companies telling us that if we hurt or feel less than optimal, all we need to do is take this drug or that drug and we will feel fine and we will be healthy. The absence of pain or *feeling well* is not health or *wellth*! As I have said, and will continue to tell you, pain is a sign that you are alive. The only way to feel no pain is to be dead or to live your life so doped up that you don't even notice that you've allowed your dreams to die and that you are slowly dying, too! This is not health or *wellth*! This is not healthy or *wellthy*!

The only way to see our lives as they really are is to turn on the light of truth and recognize what is there and deal with it. My motto has become, "It is what it is. No excuse, no guilt, no shame, no blame; it just is." So what do we do with what is? It is not "what is" but what *we do* with "what is" that will move us into the life we were born to live, into the life of "what can be." It's not about how it happened, always asking, "Why, why, why?" The better question is, "Why not turn it around and write my story the way I see it?" Often, we get so caught up in what is and why things are the way they are, that we never get past our pain and into our health and *wellth*.

Again, what are you afraid of? Where are you? What do you desire? What is it that you are willing to do right now? Are you willing to take responsibility? Are you willing to forgive yourself and others?

Don't waste your pain.
Use it to recover and restore.

Pain (physical or otherwise) is not the problem; focusing on the pain is! What is causing the pain, and what are you willing to do to remove it from your life, are more zillion-dollar questions. Remember, it is what it is…and it's *all good*! Don't waste your pain. Don't cover it up. Don't deny that it exists. Use it to recover and restore. No one else is responsible for your health, *wellth*, and happiness. Isn't that great news? It is if you *know* it!

To be "in the know" is "to possess confidential information"[4]; "confidential" is "entrusted with confidences"[5]; "confidence" is "TRUST, RELIANCE"[6]; and "a reliable [responsible] messenger brings healing."[7]

When you become responsible, you begin to heal. Since you're reading and answering the questions in this book, you are already healing (and you may not have even known you needed to heal). I love that! By the way, it's okay for you to love it, too. ☺

That voice of hope inside of you is calling out to you right now. Be answerable to the call and you will discover your answers and have a valuable life worth celebrating. I promise.

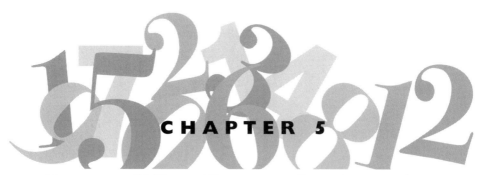

CHAPTER 5

Step #5: Be a Celebrity

Did you know?

*The more you are grateful for,
the more you will have to be grateful for.*

Celebrity: "1. the state of being celebrated : RENOWN 2. a celebrated person"[1]

Are you celebrating yourself, your life, and those in it? When you give thanks and appreciate where you are on your way to where you're going, you get there a whole lot happier. Appreciation adds so much more value and worth to your existence. Let me ask you, what makes a celebrity a celebrity? People do! If we, as a whole, didn't value a celebrity's contributions, that person wouldn't be a celebrity.

It's also quite interesting to learn how celebrities got to the place in life that they now enjoy. Most have been through some stuff—and I mean some stuff!

We've all been through stuff. I've been through some major stuff. But I don't like to call it "stuff" because stuff doesn't seem to describe it like a four-letter word would. So let's just use the four-letter word that defines it best: L-I-F-E. That's right; life is filled with stuff and when we accept it, we can usually get through the stuff a whole lot quicker.

During a time in my life when I was going through a very tough battle, the entire process shifted once I decided to celebrate, give thanks, and praise God regardless of the circumstances (the "stuff"). In those defining moments, we can all become a legend in our own lives—a celebrity!

Seriously, there is always something to be thankful for, even if it's simply in knowing that you have the ability to decide what you'll be thankful for. Years ago, I learned about Pike Place Market in Seattle, Washington. It's a world-famous fish market whose employees realized they, too, could make a difference. They wanted to make people happy, so they decided to be world famous (because people act differently when they are being world famous). They made the choice to take a "have to" and make it a "get to." They didn't want their ordinary to remain ordinary, but extraordinary. This decision has allowed them to not only be world famous, but highly influential around the world. Charthouse Learning, a company based in Minnesota, recognized their uniqueness and created a simple, yet profound, four-step process based on their world-famous work philosophy that has transformed companies and individuals around the globe. One of these steps encompasses the value of attitude.

Choosing your attitude creates the powerful realization that no longer can anyone make you mad, sad, glad, ungrateful, or anything else. Instead, you get to choose the meanings you give to the things that occur in your life. (Remember from Step #4: Do not come to a conclusion that does not serve you.) For example, you can choose to be mad. It's your right (I suppose). But you do not have to stay that way. The choice is yours.

You are the only one in control of your attitude.

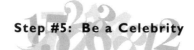

Right now, you have the power to choose to be thankful, no matter how negative your circumstances may be. You are the only one in control of your attitude. *Did you know that?* If you choose anything but a positive attitude, at least give yourself credit for being responsible for choosing that attitude! Once you realize this power, and begin living Step #4 (Be Answerable), you'll discover that taking responsibility for where you are and who you are right now is the most powerful step to getting where you want to be and being who you truly are.

If you are one hundred pounds overweight, give thanks that you have the power to release that weight. If you are having a hard time moving around due to physical pain, give thanks that you can move at all. If you have been diagnosed with cancer or another disease, give thanks that your body has a greater capacity to heal than you've ever imagined. If you have been betrayed by someone you once loved and trusted, give thanks that it is possible to forgive and love again. If you don't like certain aspects of your body, give thanks for the parts you do appreciate. (And if you don't like what you see, give thanks that you can see at all. ☺) To see things from a more thankful perspective, take a moment and imagine what life would be like without a specific body part you dislike. It might be the size of your butt, for example. Imagine if you didn't have one…where would you sit? How would you _____? (*Just kidding!*) How about this: maybe you don't like the way your thighs look. What would life be like if you had no legs at all?

A leg to stand on

I watched a documentary one time about a brilliant, beautiful, young lady whose leg was amputated at a very young age. This did not stop her from becoming a world-class triathlete, living her dreams, and fulfilling her destiny. In the interview, she said she really had a hard time when people made excuses, especially for not exercising when they had the body parts to do it. She said she would have given anything for the legs that someone else had chosen not to put to use, all because of some lame excuse! (I bet she wouldn't have complained about a less-than-perfect-looking leg if she'd had it either. Somehow, her story just puts things into perspective, doesn't it?)

Seriously, the time *is now* to stop complaining and start celebrating. Celebrate and give thanks for what you've been given. There is so very much to be thankful for—so much! Until you can be thankful for what you have, you won't get more of what you desire, I promise you that.

Do you know how I know this? I believe that even if you get more, you will likely not even recognize it. After a while, people tend to stop noticing what they already have; take their potential, for example. Is your potential waiting to be recognized? Until you recognize and give thanks for it, chances are, no one else will either. My former pastor, Pastor Randy, used to say, "Opportunities sit by quietly, just waiting to be recognized." Right here, right now, you have an opportunity to recognize and give thanks for your life and your health!

When you decide to start celebrating them, you will begin to experience them. And when you experience them, you will have health (and *wellth*)....for life. Are you protesting, "But what if this? What if that?" The "ifs" are what life is all about. Life contains "if"! It's up to you to determine what you're going to do with "if." Perhaps add L and E to make LifE, and then replace "if" with O and V to add some LOVE! When you begin to love your life, this is when your life will grow, and you'll experience more satisfaction, abundance, *wellth*, and more to love than you ever imagined!

Add a little love to your heart

You may be saying, "But my life sucks, and there is nothing in my life that I love." If that is you, then I want you to stop reading right now and do an exercise with me. In fact, even if you totally love your life (which I hope you do), you will benefit greatly from doing this simple exercise.

Go get a paper and pen. I want you to write down everything in your life that you love. Seriously, do yourself a favor and do it right now. I want you to set a timer for eleven minutes and write down as many things as you can. On your mark…get set…go!

I did this years ago, and it became a huge blessing in my life. I called it my love journal. I wrote down everything I could think of, including the feeling of wearing new socks. If it were up to me, I'd put a new pair of socks on my feet every single day. There is just something special about that feeling of a new pair of socks, don't you think? ☺ And in your life, there is definitely something or someone you can love right now!

Okay, how was it? Was it hard to stop at eleven minutes? Then go ahead and keep writing. Don't let me stop you.

For years, I have talked about my love journal when I speak to audiences, large or small. You can call your journal a love journal or a celebrity journal—they're both the same thing. They're all about recognizing and celebrating the blessings in your life. If you do that, the blessings will increase, I promise.

Now, before we go on to Step #6, I need to ask you a very important question. Did you include yourself on your list? If you did, you're ready to go on to Step #6. If not, please, please, please do not take another step. Until you are one of your biggest fans (Be a Celebrity), you are not ready to go to the next step. You can be both a humble fan and a humble celebrity! Do yourself a gigantic favor and grab another piece of paper, because you're about to experience a breakthrough that will not only set you free, but will help you see that you are extremely valuable!

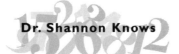

Sealed with a kiss

I want you to sit down for the next eleven minutes, or more if necessary, and write yourself a love letter. Are you saying, "What? That's crazy!" Perhaps, but what's wrong with crazy? One day I looked up the word "crazy" and discovered it's a synonym of "freak." Stay with me here; this is going to make brilliant sense in a moment. Another word for "freak" is the word "caprice." When I looked up the word "caprice," it said "CAPRICCIO." Of course I had to see what that meant, and this is what I discovered: "an instrumental piece in free form usually lively in tempo and brilliant in style."[2] How's that for being crazy? Have you ever noticed, it seems as though the crazy people are the ones who are always laughing and having a great time? How would you like to laugh more? Have a good time? Have fun? Be lively in tempo and brilliant in style? Have greater health (and *wellth*)…for life? Then it's time to do something that seems a little crazy. I promise you, this will make more sense as we go along.

Here is one thing I would like to suggest before you start. With all due respect to both genders, I have found that love seems to be the most important thing for women. It seems as though, through popular study, research, and experience, respect is the biggest deal for men. My opinion is that whether you are female or male, love and respect are both important. Therefore, if you're a woman, write yourself a letter of love and respect; and if you're a man, write yourself a letter of respect and love. Okay?

We'll talk again once you are done.

Today is the day to get out of the box, because let's face it, our boxes are taking us to the grave.

Crazy for you

This exercise may have seemed crazy because it was something you'd never done before. Hey, I assure you, if you want to get somewhere you've never been, you have to do things you've never done, right? Right!

It is time to get outside your normal, familiar way of thinking about things. Today is the day to get out of the box, because let's face it, our boxes are taking us to the grave. If you want to experience health (and *wellth*) for life, getting out of your box is vital!

Are you ready for this? This is the better part of crazy that I was talking about when I promised you this would get better: Stand in front of a mirror and read your letter out loud to yourself. Once you've done this, I want you to do yourself a favor. Do it once more, but this time, read it louder! I suggest that you continue to do this as often as you need to, until it becomes comfortable and your new "normal."

Crazy? Or is it crazy to expect to be your best when you don't even love or respect yourself? That self-defeating expectation is what's insane. Quite honestly, that is a huge conflict and stumbling block to living your best life right now. If you can settle this issue within yourself once and for all, not only will you live with much more ease, but a lot less dis-ease. Seriously!

Giving thanks is about celebrating, and that which you celebrate grows. Today is your day to celebrate your life. Give thanks for yourself and for the amazing life you're living.

As I picture you standing in front of your mirror, saying all of those amazing, empowering, grateful things about that wonderful person you see, I'm reminded of something that has happened to me more times than I can count when I've looked in the mirror.

Gratefully yours!

Approximately seven years ago, I finally saw a dermatologist for a sore on the side of my nose that just would not heal. After a biopsy, I was told that I had skin cancer. "Are you kidding me?" I thought. "How could I have cancer? Yes, I have blonde hair and fair skin, but I thought I was totally healthy."

"Would I still have a nose?" I thought.

After hearing the fact that I had skin cancer, I was scared. I thought, "What would it take to get rid of it? Would they need to cut into my face? Would I have a scar? What were my options?" At first, I wanted to do something about it immediately, so I saw a dermatologist who specialized in a technique that would remove the cancer by cutting back a flap of my skin, excising the cancer, and then stitching back the skin to, hopefully, leave a minimal scar. His plan was to continue to cut and send tissue samples to the pathology department until he had removed all traces of the skin cancer. "But what if they have to cut a lot of skin out of my nose? Would I still have a nose?" I thought.

I looked at my nose in the mirror and thought, "My nose isn't perfect, but it is *my* nose and I don't want to lose it." I had so many questions; there were so many unknowns.

The more I thought about it, the less peaceful I became. Contemplating my options, I thought, "Maybe they have some magic ointment I can just put on it and the cancer will go away." I knew that I didn't want to take any medication because the last thing my body needed was to be bombarded by a bunch of chemicals.

All of these thoughts, including my lack of peace about cutting into my face and using medication (as well as my hopeful optimism), led me to seek a supernatural healing for seven years. It was quite a journey!

Over the years, I tried several natural so-called cures and each time I was disappointed and discouraged. One natural remedy actually left my skin looking worse than ever—the sore grew bigger! I had been very hopeful that the gauze soaked in a brown stinky tincture that I bandaged to my nose each night would make a difference. It made a difference, but not the difference I'd hoped for. It was worse than ever, and now it hurt, too! Yikes!

I traveled the country seeking men and women of God who seemed to have an impressive track record for praying for those in need of healing and getting it. After hearing about a revival going on down in Florida, one night at midnight I booked a flight for a 6:00 a.m. departure out of Tulsa and a return flight at 6:00 a.m. the day after. I just knew that God could heal me. Once again, there was no sign of the healing that I'd hoped for, but I continued to be hopeful and I still knew that God could heal me. I just didn't know when.

At times I got very scared, because even though I believed that God could, my fear would cause me to wonder if in fact He would. For seven years, I would look in the mirror and put my hand up to my nose and pray for a miracle; yet, there was never a manifestation of the healing I was praying for.

That little voice inside my head (you know the one—that mean little voice of fear and doubt that sounds so authoritative and confident) kept telling me that eventually I would have to have it cut out. And worse yet, because I'd waited so long for "my God to heal it" (imagine both hands up with the fingers sarcastically doing the quote thing) but He hadn't, they would now have to remove half my nose and leave me scarred and disfigured for life. Then I would think, "But people have nose jobs, so perhaps I'll just get a nose job when that happens and my nose will look better than ever. Or not." Then I would wonder how much it would cost to have plastic surgery. Would I be able to afford it? Then I would imagine standing in front of a large group of people telling my story, but the only difference would be that I'd have to tell them, "God *is* a healer, but in this case, for whatever reason, He just didn't heal me." How would that make me look? More importantly, how would that make God look? I didn't want to look bad physically or spiritually, but I definitely didn't want God to look bad! All these thoughts went through my head off and on for years, but especially more as time went on.

I even began to contemplate putting a drug on it. A friend of mine had used a special "hand-me-down" prescription ointment that was left over from her mom's skin cancer treatment. *(Please note: Do not ever use another person's prescription, especially one that is old. By the way, it is not only extremely dangerous, but it's illegal!)* Although it took away the skin cancer, it caused the entire side of her face to blister up and ooze with nastiness, and it made her eye red, watery, and blurry. She had to wear an eye patch for days. I imagined how I would look as I sat in front of my patients with a red open wound on the side of my nose and face, wearing an eye patch and explaining that their bodies were designed by God to be self-healing. I just couldn't see this being the route that God had for me.

The Bible says I should be led by peace.

Don't get me wrong; I believe God can use doctors and He can use medicine at times to save lives, as well as to treat skin cancer, but I just couldn't accept that route as God's best plan for me. The Bible says I should be led by peace, and no matter how much I wanted a quick fix, I just did not have peace about doing anything invasive.

Then in the spring of 2009, as I was preparing for a mission trip to India—one that I had anticipated and desired in my heart for a decade—I prayed once again for a miracle healing for my skin. (I was so excited about the incredible opportunity and being able to finally travel to India to serve God by serving those in need!)

The day before I left, this thought hit me: "Yes, I'm going to India to serve, but I believe that God has something for *me* to receive while I'm there, as well."

I wondered what it would be, and then it came to me, "I'm going to get the healing I've been seeking for years! *God healed the lepers' skin, and He can heal my skin, too.* I just know it!" Then I prayed, and after reminding God that He can heal leprosy (like He needed reminding ☺), I asked Him once again to pretty-pretty please heal my skin!

I left for India very hopeful that I would return cancer free!

Once we arrived in India, my hope began to build. I was traveling with a powerful group of chiropractors, pastors, and men and women of great faith; people who had witnessed countless miracles. On this trip, we witnessed blind people seeing, lame people walking, and deaf people hearing—for the first time in their lives! I was so caught up in the anticipation of all that God was going to do for people that I didn't think about what He was going to do for me; that is, until I was told we were going to visit a leper colony!

"What! A leper colony?" I thought.

"What! A leper colony?" I thought. I didn't even think there was such a thing in this day and age. Little did I know. I wondered what we would see and experience when we got there. Then I started to feel a little (okay, a lot!) scared. I wondered, "Is leprosy contagious? What were we going to do for them? Pray?" Then I was reminded of the talk I'd had with God before I left. "God, you can heal the lepers. Please heal them and pretty-pretty please heal me!" All of a sudden, I wasn't so afraid, plus I knew that our leader wouldn't take us to a leper colony if it were dangerous. Then God reminded me that our team had prayed several times before leaving for safety and protection, so I knew I had nothing to worry about. But just to be on the safe side, I wouldn't touch anything or anyone. Or so I thought.

What I experienced at that leper colony was one of the most divine, humbling experiences I have ever had. Those people with leprosy were so happy, so full of joy! When I looked into their eyes, I saw nothing but the love of God and the hope of a nation. I was so moved and absolutely inspired; and oh…did I mention, humbled?

They sang to us, and a few told their stories about how God had led them to this colony and how much the local ministry had helped them. Even though they were missing limbs, they weren't lacking in abundant love, gratitude, and appreciation.

Everything was going well as I enjoyed them from a short distance, until all of a sudden, (have you ever noticed that the "all of a suddens" in life tend to impact us the most?) I heard one of the other chiropractors saying, "We are going to adjust them." For a split second, I thought I heard him wrong, but then "all of a sudden" my head stopped thinking and my heart started serving, and I was no longer afraid. I was totally moved with compassion and gratitude for the honor of being able to lay my hands on these mighty men and women and pray for them, as I administered a specific chiropractic adjustment. (Note: For those of you who don't know what I mean, I placed my hands on their necks and gave a very gentle thrust, not only to move the misaligned vertebrae in their upper necks or lower backs—whatever they needed—but to free up their nervous systems to function optimally.) It was absolutely amazing! They were very grateful for our care and I think even more grateful for our touch! I have never been so humbled!

When I left the leper colony, I couldn't quit thinking about what had just happened. Then I began to talk to God about it. "Please heal them, Lord. Bless them and comfort them," I pleaded. "Lord, I want to love you like that! Thank you for giving me the opportunity to be used by you in such a way, to touch those wonderful people who love you so much, and whom you deeply love!"

The next night we were praising and worshipping God as we ministered to a crowd of thousands. I was completely engulfed in the presence of the Lord, just oozing with gratitude and love, when I asked God once more, "Please heal my skin."

Then I heard Him say, not in an audible voice, but in the kind of voice that's much louder than that—a voice from deep within—"Do not ask me that again."

"What! Did God just tell me not to ask Him that again?" Quite honestly, for a moment I was a little irritated with what I'd just heard; not unlike a teenage girl would feel if her dad bluntly said, "Do not ask me that again" after she'd been begging for hours. In my case, for years!

"Just give thanks."

Once I got over my moment of offense, I quickly thought, "That must mean that it's finished, it's done, I'm healed! If He doesn't want me to ask again, it must mean I won't have to!" I was so excited. Then I asked Him, "Then what should I do?" He so beautifully responded, "Just give thanks." Wow! What an overwhelming moment; one that I will never forget!

So I agreed with God and began to do just that. "Thank you so much, God! Thank you! Thank you! Thank you!" Then I simply requested that He give me a manifestation of the healing before I left India, even if it was just a little sign. I continued in praise and worship, and that night, I saw many people healed of such things as deafness, cancer, and blindness, as well as thousands give their lives to Christ. It was a miraculous evening, to say the least.

The next morning as I was getting ready for the day, I was putting on makeup even though it was so hot that I sweated it off almost immediately. I felt God tell me to stop covering the area on the side of my nose with makeup, as I had done for so many years. Since I already had it on, I told Him that I wouldn't cover it up anymore. (Seriously, thinking back, He had to have been rolling His eyes at me! Like I couldn't have just wiped it off right then? Dang! ☺)

By the time I left India, my skin was changing. It was looking a lot less red, and smaller. (If it had been covered with makeup, I wouldn't have been able to see the changes.) Even my friend Alicia thought it looked better. I was so grateful and so very hopeful!

Upon returning home, I would like to say that my skin continued to look better, but it didn't. In fact, it began to look worse and seemed to be getting bigger. Several times I stopped myself just before the words "God, please heal my skin!" came out of my mouth. It was especially hard every morning as I looked in the mirror expecting to see change for the better, but seeing what appeared to be change for the worse. I wanted to cover it with makeup, but I didn't.

When I wanted to ask again, but didn't, I just thanked Him. I thanked Him that He was manifesting the healing and then I just thanked Him for who He was. I was doing what He asked, or so I thought. "Could there be more?" I wondered.

One day I thought, "What would I do if I were really grateful for healthy skin and a healthy body?" The more I thought about it, I realized that one of the greatest ways that I could show God how grateful I was would be to take the very best possible care of my body.

So often, we say we appreciate something or someone, but then we don't act as though we really do. If I were really grateful for my healthy body, would I feed it sugar? Lots of sugar? Especially when I've read countless times how cancer feeds on sugar! Would I stand in front of the mirror and say mean things about the way I look? Would I take the vitamins that I know help nourish my skin and my body? Would I exercise the strength that God has given me by doing activities that exercise my body, especially the ones that I love the most? If I didn't have legs that worked, would I long to get back the many days when I just didn't feel like exercising and now wish that I could?

I decided to take my self-care to a whole new level. I purposed in my mind and heart to show God my appreciation by caring for my body the best way that I could. I began to meet with a friend of mine who used to be an oncologist, but who now is a natural health expert. I asked him to hold me accountable to take my vitamins and do the things that I know to do to strengthen my immune system and help my body help itself. He agreed, and the accountability helped me tremendously.

The more you are grateful for, the more you will have to be grateful for.

Then one day I was having a little chat with God about it again, and this is what He told me: "Live a grateful life. The more you are grateful for, the more you will have to be grateful for."

So this is what I've done. And I can attest, grateful really equals full of great. I promise!

Not long afterward, I began to notice a change in the way my skin was looking. Once again, it was looking worse! But this time there was something different. It appeared to be bubbling out and looking a little more like a tumor, instead of a sore that just wouldn't heal. For a moment, I got scared again. ("What! A tumor?") But then I reminded myself of what God had said to me and I just thanked Him for the changes.

I told my friend about what was happening. He saw what I saw as well, although I don't think he was as convinced as I was that the change was a positive one. I told him, "You just watch; this is going to bubble out and the next thing we'll know, it'll just fall off, and only a little dent will remain." He lifted his eyebrows and cautiously agreed.

That is precisely what happened! Over the next several days, I watched it become a bigger bump on the side of my nose, and then one day, it was miraculously gone! And to this day, there is no sign of it! God healed me! (Thank you, God!)

I am so grateful! And the greatest thing I can tell you is, *He can heal you, too!*

Be grateful right where you are. Celebrate your life. Celebrate yourself. "The more you are grateful for, the more you will have to be grateful for." I didn't say it, God did. I just agree with Him, and I suggest you do the same!

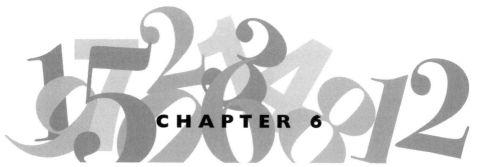

CHAPTER 6

Step #6: Be Valuably Free

Did you know?

The simplest way to let go of what was is to grab hold of what is.

When we recognize our value and begin to celebrate it, we become free to be exactly who we were created to be. This freedom allows us to let go of the control we thought we had or we attempted to have and keeps us from the control we've been under.

Let me ask you this: If you are tied to a rope, are you free? Of course not. What is the difference between being tied to a rope and holding on to a rope? The answer is the ability to let go. How about this: What if you are holding on to a rope but you think you're tied to it? How will you know if you are tied up or merely holding on? Simple; let go!

No words, actions, persuasion, or possibility can let go for you. If you have taken Steps #1-#5, then this step will be quite simple. Notice, I did not say "easy." It isn't easy because, for some reason, we tend to make this step much harder than it is. Actually, the steps leading up to this moment take the most time and energy; therefore, letting go is the simple part *if* you allow yourself to open the hand that has been tightly holding on.

(And you wonder why your muscles hurt? Whether the one in your head or the ones in your back and shoulders.)

For years, I tried to control myself and my circumstances, although not necessarily in a bad way. Regardless of my intentions, my effort to control created a "bad way" at times. Trying to control things proved to be a much harder way to get from point A to point B than it needed to be. I not only attempted to control myself and my circumstances but the results and the outcomes, too. This definitely caused a much more difficult journey than would have been necessary had I learned and practiced this step years ago.

But hey, what doesn't kill you makes you stronger, right? I say that somewhat jokingly now, but oh, it has been so very true in my life! One time I remember asking my best friend, Melly, "When is it going to stop being so hard?"

She responded, "When you're ready for it to stop being hard."

"What? Are you kidding me?" I asked. Needless to say, I didn't appreciate hearing that philosophical crap right at that moment. You see, I didn't know how to let it *not* be hard.

Once again, I thought it was something *I* had to do. What I understood her to say was that *I* needed to make it "not hard," when the truth of the matter was, I didn't really need to do anything except embrace what was and let go! That would have been the way to stop "doing hard."

I know it sounds too easy, doesn't it? Well, I'll tell you, you're right; embracing what is and letting go is not real easy, but there is a supernatural ease to it. It is definitely much easier than "doing hard." Best of all, it is quite simple, so simple that it is one of the most profound things I've ever experienced and lived to tell about. It is also infinitely easier than holding on. Trust me! ☺

Surrender is a great gift.

Letting go is not quitting or giving up; instead, I see it as surrender. Surrender is a great gift. I had been wrestling with my situation like a gold medalist Olympic Greco-Roman wrestler and I, by golly, would wear my medal with pride, come hell or high water (as my dad would say ☺).

If you've been doing the same, the problem is, that medal will eventually become a noose around your neck. You'll think you're tied to your pain and its powerlessness, when the truth is, you don't have to wear that weight any longer. And as far as being tied to it? All you need to do is bow your head and let it slip off.

When I truly put my hands in the air and gave up the fight, I won. I began to get my life back and so will you.

When I think of surrendering, I picture standing with my hands up and moving forward in peace. This is exactly what happened. It is also why the beginning of the word (and the process of) "restoration" is *rest*!

One morning while I was doing one of my very favorite things—boxing (yes, boxing!)—I experienced a great feeling of rest, and I recognized and embraced it. You're probably wondering how in the world anyone could feel restful while boxing. Well, what I have realized through many experiences is that rest doesn't have to mean lying on a sofa or in a bed trying to rejuvenate. Instead, I have experienced rest from a state of grateful ease and from embracing the moment that I was in. That morning, I was feeling so happy and so free! That's always what I feel when I'm boxing or engaging in forms of exercise that I absolutely love, like running or teaching a group-fitness class. But that morning I was feeling something that made such an impression on me that I want to share it with you.

When I tell people I love to box, often they tilt their heads and give me *that look* that says, "*You?* You're supposed to be this nurturing healer who is gentle and loving. You're a chiropractor! How can boxing be good for your spine?" I explain to them that we don't box each other in the head and usually, I'm the one doing most of the punching (unless I'm in the ring with Carl ☺), and it is not violent or aggressive; at least not for me. It's quite simply a moment to exercise my strength and practice my technique, as well as to sharpen my focus. It is absolutely wonderful. Often when I am punching and I start to feel a little out of breath or somewhat tired, I ask myself, "If this was the last time I could do this, how would I box today?" It always helps me punch harder, move quicker, and love every minute of it even more.

As I punched very hard that morning I thought, "Wow, this almost seems like I'm letting out some aggression or something, but I'm not." Then I was reminded of something that happened a couple weeks earlier that had the potential to make me feel very aggressive, but I was so thankful that it hadn't at all, because I had chosen to let it go. I believe that letting it go allowed me to experience that beautiful rest and valuable freedom that morning in the boxing ring.

What happened a couple weeks earlier? I'm so glad you asked! Let's call it a valuable life lesson, one that I will never forget, and one that, oddly, I am very grateful for.

Lessons from a thief

I was in my office on a conference call with a gentleman regarding the vision I have for my personal finances. Interestingly enough, when that gentleman asked me about my current insurance policies, including home, auto, and health, I told him that I was very likely overinsured. He responded, "I will have you speak with another one of my associates about analyzing your insurance needs." Nonetheless, I was on the phone with that associate when I got a call from my frantic neighbor telling me that she had gone home for lunch and noticed that my front door had been kicked in! She said it appeared as though I had been burglarized!

"What? Are you kidding me? What about my dog, did they take my dog?" That was all I could think about. Nothing else mattered to me at that moment except the whereabouts of my sweet little dog, as well as an insurmountable gratitude for the fact that my daughter was out of town visiting family when the burglary occurred. (Thank God!)

After informing my neighbor to call the police, I told my business advisor that I would call him back another time, and I drove home as quickly as I could. I have never prayed so much in what seemed to be the longest fifteen minutes of my life! My thoughts were not on what they stole from me, but how much I loved my dog and how much I didn't want to have to tell my daughter that her dog was missing.

As I entered my home, I was overcome with intense gratitude upon finding my dog safe and sound. But then I was overwhelmed with great sadness because of the state my house was in. Every drawer, cupboard, closet, and room had been sifted through and my things were everywhere! Two police officers stood there amidst the mess. I wasn't sure what the thieves had taken. All I knew was that I was missing that happy, safe, sacred, secure feeling that always embraced me when I entered my home.

The thief or thieves had gone through every box that looked like it could contain something of value. They took all of my rings (and there were a lot of them—I just love fun, funky rings, some expensive and some not—but all of them were very valuable to me, especially the inexpensive rare finds from travels around the world), and several expensive pieces of jewelry. That was it!

Just a little side note: I found it interesting that they didn't take anything except rings and a few pieces of expensive jewelry. They did not take my camera, laptop, flat-screen TV, or anything else. It made me realize that even crooks have a specialty. They choose what it is they are going for and they stick to it. As weird as it sounds, it made me appreciate the value of choosing what to focus on and doing it big. If they had tried to take everything, they would have likely gotten away with nothing! So let's just call that a little nugget of value that my thief gave me.

It reminds me of another nugget I heard a friend say years ago: "Just because you can, doesn't mean you should." This has helped me stay focused several times in my life when I've been surrounded by many opportunities. I've learned that specificity and timing are everything when it comes to getting the results we are looking for.

The big lesson I learned that day goes something like this: It seems as though we as humans are so concerned about our valuables that we place them in little boxes inside bigger boxes and store them up high on a shelf we consider to be a safe place, and there they sit. But are they really safe? The possessions of value the thief didn't steal were those I had with me that day.

As valuable human beings, are we safe in the boxes we live in? Isn't it time to start living outside of your box? The greatest way to do that is by becoming truly free. It is time to let go so you get to go wherever it is you desire to be. It is time to be valuably free!

How? By putting up your arms and surrendering! (Perhaps this is exactly what that thief will do when they find him with all my stuff!) Stop right now and turn yourself in; get out of your box, knowing that your greatest value is not how much you have in your boxes, but what you have on the innermost part of you—the most valuable gift of all!

The only thing you have that cannot be stolen is that which is inside of you.

The only safety and security we have is what comes from the inside, out. Real rest and freedom come from within and no man or woman can take them from you; they can only have them if you choose to give them away.

As I was "resting" in the boxing ring that morning, I felt grateful that I didn't give away my joy by being bitter or unforgiving toward the individual (or individuals) who stole from me. Best of all, I had begun to sense that safe, secure feeling in my home again. Once I realized that my safety had never been compromised, because my daughter, dog, and I had in fact been kept safe, I was so grateful! I truly believe that somehow, some way, I will get my jewelry back.

Webster's New American Dictionary defines "surrender" as "to give oneself up or yield." It also says that when we yield we "bring forth by natural process; bear (as fruit) produce." Isn't that beautiful? This letting go is essential for bearing (or yielding) the fruit you were designed to bear, and in this way, becoming the person you were designed to be.

Whatever it is that has gotten you tied up, tied down, or torn up—it is time to let go once and for all.

It's time to fly

Ever since I could remember, I had been fascinated with the idea of skydiving. It sat on my so-called "Someday I Will" list, until one day, I did it. It was the year 2000, and I had just been through a major life transition (divorce). Those of us who have been through such an experience have so much to let go of—so much hurt, anger, disappointment, failure. We need help in forgiving others, as well as ourselves. Skydiving seemed like the perfect way to deal with the new cards I'd been given. (By the way, if you are currently dealing with heartache and divorce, be encouraged! What may seem like an absolute dead end is just a detour and you *will* get to where you've always desired to go as long as you keep looking and moving ahead. Trust me! I've been where you are, so I know there is light at the end of the tunnel, and life after divorce. I promise! These twelve steps will help you get through it, just as they did for me.)

About twelve people from my church were also interested in doing this unthinkable feat—jumping out of a plane at fourteen thousand feet above the earth! This was the opportunity I had been looking for. I called my dear friend, Melly, and we decided to jump together.

After anticipating such a thrill for so many years, it was hard to believe it was finally going to happen. We drove to a place in Wisconsin that was out in the middle of nowhere in the midst of a lot of farmland. I don't know what I'd been expecting, but I guess it made sense to land in an open field, rather than jump into a bunch of rolling hills and trees.

My heart was beginning to wonder, "What was it going to be like? Would I be scared? Would it be as awesome as I hoped it would be? Would it help me move past my present situation and into a life of fear-less victory? Would my parachute even open?" (Yes, I hate to admit it, but that question did flash through my head a couple times. Yikes!) "Of course it would," I thought. But just in case, "Dear Lord, please help my chute to open and help me land without whiplashing my neck," I prayed.

Next thing I knew, our jump masters were picking out our jumpsuits. I was given a bright pink one; Mel was given a bright yellow one. (I wanted a yellow one, but this should really have been the least of my concerns; I was about to jump out of a plane traveling fourteen thousand feet above the ground! ☺) I reasoned that as long as I had a parachute that worked, it didn't even have to match my jumpsuit.

We had our skintight suits on and had received specific instructions on what to do and what not to do. Our jump masters had on our reliable parachutes (whether they matched our outfits or not) and we were ready to load the plane. "What!" I thought. "This is really happening!" My heart was pounding faster and louder…

We got into a plane that looked nothing like planes I'd ever been in. No carpet, no restrooms, and no flight attendants promised us a safe and comfortable flight! I just remembered seeing a lot of bare steel and thinking, "I hope I don't have to pee when I get up there."

Then it was time. The door opened and we were instructed to stand up (along with the jump master who was attached to our back) and move toward the open door of the plane. "Oh my goodness, what am I doing?" I thought. My videographer who would jump just a moment ahead of me had already launched out and it was my time...

A friend of mine who had jumped several times had given me a gift certificate for a videographer to jump with me. She instructed me to be sure I smiled the whole time.

"Why?" I'd asked her.

"Because if you don't keep the muscles in your face contracted with a smile, the skin on your face will do all sorts of crazy, not-so-attractive kinds of contortions while the wind is whipping against it, as you fall very fast from the plane you just jumped out of. That's why!" The focus was all about making sure I looked good on my video, I guess. At that moment, what I looked like really didn't seem to be a priority!

"OK, I will do my best to try to look good ☺," I thought. Oh, and I was supposed to keep my eyes on my videographer the whole time. (As if I was going to be able to find him flying out there. He had already jumped and I was still in the plane!)

Standing in front of the open door, the ground looked so far away. Suddenly, the notion of this being a cool thing to do didn't seem so cool. Very cold and windy, yes, but nothing noble or nice! "What the heck am I doing?" was the only thing I heard in my head. I can assure you, I wasn't thinking about the color of my jumpsuit, finding my videographer, or smiling for the camera!

I jumped and all I could think of was that I was falling and that I was completely and absolutely out of control! What had I just done? The feeling of *falling fast* was overwhelming! The rush of fear that came over me was unlike anything I'd ever experienced or would choose to experience again. Needless to say, I was totally freaked out and free-falling to the ground from almost three miles high, *very, very fast*! Once again, I did not think about smiling or making a great video. In fact, my videographer was nowhere in sight. (Oh, and did I mention how *very* fast I was falling to the ground that was rapidly approaching!)

Then all of a sudden, there he was right in front of me and I was no longer falling. I was flying, and it was the most outrageous, beautiful thing I had ever felt! In that moment, I was as free as a bird and nothing mattered except, of course, smiling for my cameraman! ☺ I will never forget that spectacular feeling of flying as time stood still. Awesome!

Then another "all of a sudden" happened (you have to appreciate the "suddenlies" in life). My jump master (I forgot he was on my back) tapped my shoulder and I braced myself for the next step. I crossed my arms and tucked my chin as our chute opened and we were forcefully pulled from a horizontal, flying position to a vertical one, not unlike a fish being pulled out of the water. Wow, that sure was an abrupt finish to what seemed like the most incredible moment I had ever encountered.

The parachute finally fully opened (I knew it would ☺) and I was no longer flying, but instead, floating like a butterfly with only the sound of peace filling the air! It was by far the most quiet, serene moment I had ever been blessed to be a part of. All I could do was praise God and thank Him for His greatness and all that He is! Nothing else seemed to matter; just He and me in that moment. Everything seemed so simple and so clear. I felt no worry, no fear, no anxiety, no hurt, and no pain. Besides giving birth to my daughter, it was by far the greatest moment of my life! I am absolutely convinced that heaven is going to feel like this!

> *You will go from fearing, to falling, to flying,*
> *to floating; and the freedom you will embrace*
> *is absolutely heaven on earth!*

This is exactly what happens when you face your fears, locate yourself, know what you desire, take responsibility, celebrate, and let go! You will go from fearing, to falling, to flying, to floating; and the freedom you will embrace is absolutely heaven on earth!

When you let go, you will allow yourself to discover possibilities you never knew existed, and the life you were born to live. Try it—I dare you!

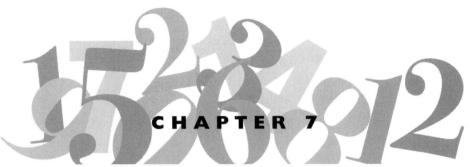

CHAPTER 7

Step #7: Be Question-able

Did you know?

Your life is the answer to the questions you ask.

Have you noticed that every step so far has included asking questions—great questions? Great questions lead to great answers. Since you've taken Step #4 (Be Answerable), you are in a perfect position to ask as many questions as you would like because you are *answerable*, right?

One of my coaches used to ask me, "What is the plural of ask?" Then he'd say, "Ask means ask, no matter how many times you ask." Ask for whatever it is you desire, and keep asking. It really is that simple.

If you want to experience health and *wellth* for life, you need to be question-able. *Ask!* Ask questions, ask for help, ask, ask, and ask. We have not, because we ask not. Whether we ask one time or a thousand times, all we need to do is ask.

The power of questions

My dear friend, Noah St. John, talks about the incredible power that lies within the simple, yet profound questions we ask ourselves. He calls them Afformations. (No, that is not a typo; I didn't intend to write affirmations.)   Afformations are like affirmations, but are questions that we ask ourselves versus statements we say about ourselves.   For example, a typical affirmation may be, "I am so healthy and *wellthy.*" An Afformation would be, "Why am I so healthy and *wellthy?*" I suggest that you read his book, *The Secret Code of Success,* to learn more about how he discovered Afformations and their dynamic power.

I have known Noah for years, have trained with him on several occasions, and helped him with a little book that he wrote years ago called, *The Great Little Wellness Book of Afformations.*   I have seen the power of Afformations work powerfully in his life, as well as in my own life, but still, I so often fail to even think to ask and afform.   Why is that?   I'm convinced it's because asking and afforming are so simple, they seem too good to be true; I guess I probably take them for granted.

Two years ago, I was thinking about Afformations when I decided, "What the heck, I'm going to start afforming again and just see what happens."   So I did.   My new Afformations were: **"Why am I so rich?"** (*My income was down and it seemed like I had more bills than money.*) **"Why am I so healthy?"** (*I was still waiting for the manifestation of my miraculous healing from skin cancer.*) **"Why am I so fit?"**   (*I had gained a little weight after my first trip to India and was feeling a little out of shape. Maybe it had something to do with the jet lag and waking up in the middle of the night and eating for two weeks straight. Yikes!*) **"Why am I so wealthy?"** (*I just threw that in there, because who doesn't want to be wealthy—the more I have, the more I have to give!*) **"Why am I so free?"** (*This had been my desire as long as I can remember, especially after my divorce. At times, no matter how good things were in my life, I just didn't feel free, especially during my year of hectic busyness while desperately trying to find rest.*) **"Why am I so happy?"** (*I was happy, but I wanted to be "so happy"!*) **"Why am I so successful?"** (*My life was so hectic and lacking in freedom that I didn't feel very successful, even though from the outside looking in, I appeared* *successful.*) **"Why am I so pretty?"** (*I just threw that one in there because I always want to look young and pretty or at least think I look young and pretty* ☺, *especially as I get older—without Botox or surgery, by the way. Seriously, I've had to do Step #1 about this many times because a fear of looking old has often tried to come on me. Now don't get me wrong; I know several older people who are absolutely gorgeous, but who knows what I'm going to look like when I'm 70, 90, and 111? Yes, I plan to live until I am 111! Will my skin still fit me? I have fear about this, so now I even do an Afformation of "Why is my skin so healthy, firm, and young looking?"*☺ *I admit it, I want to be pretty and I don't want to look old! Call me vain, but I am serious and I told you I would tell you the truth, and that is the truth. Seriously, admit it; you've probably thought about this, too. I can't be the only one!*)

So I did my new Afformations for I don't even know how long. Then, I didn't think about them again until I was going through some old videos I had recorded. I came across the one in which I was saying those Afformations and it reminded me once again of how absolutely amazing the power of asking the right questions really is!

The video was an old nspirer video. (No, that isn't a typo. I do a video blog called "*the nspirer.*") It's about lessons that life gives me, and it's simply life as I see it. So I refer to it as "*the nspirer…inspiring minds that want to grow and hearts that want to know.*"

In the video I was talking about the power of the questions we ask ourselves, and I shared my Afformations. Oh my goodness, I was absolutely amazed! Let me tell you why. Ever since finding that video, I've been reflecting on all God has done for me and I am so grateful. I thank God for everything He has done, and I thank Him for Afformations as well!

Since using those Afformations, the following has happened:

1. Eleven days after I made that old video, I met the man who is now my husband, and I wasn't even thinking about a relationship when I created my new Afformations. (*By the way, he is the*

123

most incredible man I have ever met and truly has brought so much richness into my life. We make each other laugh…a lot. We share the same mission and purpose, and are touching the world together. He has definitely turned my "happy" into "so happy"!)

2. I am totally healed of skin cancer!

3. I am back to my fit size and shape.

4. I have a new office space for a fraction of what I was previously paying.

5. My income has more than doubled and my expenses have decreased.

6. My new home is more than four times the size of my previous home.

7. I am driving a new vehicle that was given to me. Please let me explain: Probably about six months before getting my new vehicle, I was praying about my desire for one. I had a 2001 Nissan Xterra that I absolutely loved (bright yellow ☺), but it was getting old. I was discussing this with God one day when the wildest thought came to my mind: Why not just ask God to bless me with a new vehicle? I had heard of God giving people vehicles before, some of whom I knew personally, but the thought of God giving one to me had never before crossed my mind. This was probably because I figured that since I could afford to buy one, I shouldn't ask. So I thought, "What the heck, I'm going to ask and see what happens. It can't hurt to ask."

I absolutely believe in the power of asking in prayer.

I absolutely believe in the power of asking in prayer, and so I did. God is an awesome God and He wants us to *ask*, and not just when we're desperate. I really believed it could happen, but I didn't know how or when. About a month or so after I was driving my new car, suddenly it occurred to me that God had answered my prayer! Oh my goodness, I hadn't even realized that I'd forgotten to thank Him for giving me a new vehicle. So I stopped and thanked Him right then, and I continue to on a regular basis! God is *so good!*

8. I have never felt so free, happy, contented, and peaceful as I do right now. I am truly living the life of my dreams, and there is nothing better!

9. I went from having one beautiful, amazing daughter to having three!

10. I traveled around the world for the second time in a year, and God has given me opportunities to continue to do this. And I am traveling with my husband! It is truly a dream come true for me!

11. We are serving more people in my office than ever before (with less stress) and God has opened up many doors of opportunity to grow and serve, both locally and internationally! This includes being on staff at the Cancer Treatment Centers of America.

12. I have completed the very book you hold in your hands, one that I believe will touch and transform lives all over the world. This is a dream I've had for decades, and none of this would have been possible without taking the steps that I'm sharing with you today, especially this one—daring to *ask*! (*Being Question-able.*)

13. My life is full of pretty. Wherever I look, I see the beautiful life God has given me. All the health and *wellth* on the inside of me are reflecting on my outside. ☺

Please know that I've mentioned all these specific and very personal things not to impress you (I am not impressive, but God and His truth are!), but to humbly impress upon you the extraordinary power you hold within the questions you ask and the steps you take.

Thank you for reading and sharing in my celebration. If God can do it for me, He can do it for you, too. I thank God for giving us the ability to ask and to simply give thanks. ☺

God wants you to ask, because He has so much to give!

Noah St. John teaches that our subconscious minds are designed to answer the questions we ask ourselves. The answer our subconscious minds give us is reflected in the life we live, whether one of health versus sickness, life versus death, abundance versus lack, creation versus destruction. The course of our lives has everything to do with the questions we ask ourselves and others.

So many times, we ask ourselves disempowering questions such as, "Why me? Why am I so fat? Why can't I lose weight? Why doesn't anyone love me?" Our destructive list goes on and on. Instead, we could be asking, "Why not me?" (*Imagine the possibility.*) "Why am I so fit?" (*Because I exercise and eat well.*) "Why am I losing weight?" (*Because I am following the "health4life REVOLUTION!" plan and loving it.*) "Why am I so loveable?" (*Because I love myself!*)

Asking yourself the right questions is absolutely essential to a healthy, *wellthy* life, but so is your ability and willingness to ask questions of others. Asking for help is huge, especially when we ask God for help. You see, once we isolate ourselves from others and refuse to ask for help (as well as receive the help we need), we are vulnerable to the self-destructive thought processes and habits that first got us in the shape we're in. Does that make sense?

The acceptable no

The thoughts we think and the words we speak are the building blocks of the life we're living. Our thoughts become our words and, eventually, our destiny. Our tongues have the power to create or destroy ourselves and those around us. Creativity is the key to a healthy, *wellthy* life. Our thoughts and words are a creative force. We get to choose the thoughts we entertain and the words that become our domain.

> *Don't believe everything you think.*
>
> *Don't speak every thought you think.*

The other day I was driving in a town near mine when I spotted a sign in front of a business that said, "Don't believe everything you think." Wow! I had to pull over and write that one down. I would add this as well: Don't speak every thought you think.

As I said, we get to choose the thoughts we entertain. We cannot always choose the thoughts that come flying through our heads, but we do get to choose whether or not we're going to engage them—dance with them, speak them, and eventually believe them.

The next time you have a thought that comes to your mind seemingly out of nowhere, think of it as a stranger coming up and asking you to dance. You can say "Yes," or "No, thank you." And I've got news for you; no is a perfectly acceptable answer, and thank you is completely optional.

Just because someone asks, doesn't mean you have to say yes. Just because your phone rings, doesn't mean you have to answer the call. Just because you think something, doesn't mean you have to accept it, speak it, or believe it!

Did you know the thoughts you think come from the beliefs you hold? Seriously, if you're not sure you know what you believe, then spend a moment or two with your thoughts, and you will gain some insight about your beliefs. For example, if you believe you are a victim, your thoughts will usually sound something like this: "Why me? Why can't I? Why does she always get __?_ and I don't? Why can't I lose weight?"

On the other hand, if you believe (really believe) that within you is an infinite power of possibility and victory, you will think and ask questions such as: "How can I share this with others? How can I help you? What can I do today with this amazing gift?" From these questions will come words of thanksgiving and praise, and a life that will draw others to you. People will want to know what it is that makes you different. They will be curious about how you became so healthy and so *wellthy*, and you can tell them. The world is hungry for the truth and will invest their lives in search of what they believe they don't have. When you tell them they no longer need to chase after it because what they seek lies within them, imagine the impact your words will have!

The quality of our lives is in direct proportion to the quality of our relationships.

Who are you influencing, and more importantly, who is influencing you? Healthy, *wellthy* living is all about healthy relationships. I believe the quality of our lives is in direct proportion to the quality of our relationships. How healthy (*wellthy*) are you? Take a look at your relationships and you will quickly see how healthy (*wellthy*) you truly are. This includes the relationship you have with yourself, so how do you talk to yourself?

The greatest way to relate to others and yourself is by sharing what you have on the inside of you. When you do, an abundant channel will open up for you to receive what you need to grow and prosper. Sharing is essential for receiving, whether it is a simple request for help, or giving from the greatness within you. Either way, sharing gives you permission to receive the blessings you were destined to receive.

I encourage you to stop asking God, "Why me?" Instead, ask Him, "Why am I so wonderful?" He will remind you that He made you that way. Ask Him to help you recognize your blessings and share them with others. God can give you the answer to your prayers because He has already put inside you what you need to succeed. My life changed dramatically once I stopped asking "Why me?" and instead asked for wisdom and let the words of my lips be words of thanksgiving and praise.

Where there is life, there is hope for healing. Life flows from above, down, inside, and out, and that is exactly how you will heal—from above, down, inside, and out. Above (from God, then from your head/brain), down (to the rest of your body and life).

We are transformed by the renewing of our minds. How does this happen? By making a decision. You see, people think that change takes time, and that's true. Healing also takes time, but transformation happens the moment you make a decision. Healing begins in the moment of decision. The power to choose is one of the greatest gifts we've been given. We have the ability and the responsibility to choose life over death.

Because we have been created in the image of God Himself, we have the ability to speak life or death; blessings or curses. This is simply based on the words we choose to use; the words that come out of our mouths. So often, when we think about being healthy, we think about the stuff that goes *in* our mouths. Although this is very true and vitally important, even more profound is the impact our words have, not only on our bodies, but on our spirits, minds, will, and emotions. Basically, our lives!

God is the solution

For many years in my practice, I've watched countless numbers of people come into my office complaining of suffering, sickness, and disease. What has been most intriguing, although disturbing, is the fact that so many of them also confess to believe in the power of God to not only heal, but to help them live an abundant life. So why are they living so far below the level of greatness God promises?

One day I was asking God about this, and this is the revelation He gave me. The Bible says that by believing in our heart and confessing with our mouth that Jesus is Lord, we can have eternal life.[1] This is what allows us to live as believers with the promise of heaven and eternal life. That is so awesome! It's essential to do these two things to receive salvation. I get it, but what I didn't quite get until that moment of revelation is the importance of these two things for a heaven-on-earth existence while we live here on planet Earth. We believe for __?__ (whatever __?__ is for each of us), but our words do not line up with what we are believing God for. We believe that God can heal, and we believe for healing, but with our words we confess for sickness and death! The words coming out of our mouths are incongruent with what we believe. We talk about the problem while we believe that God provides the solution.

Instead of just analyzing what is coming out of our mouths, we should analyze what is in our hearts! The Bible says, "Out of the abundance of the heart the mouth speaks."[2] Perhaps we are saying that we believe something, but in reality, we actually believe something else. Perhaps we believe more in the obvious problem, instead of the not-yet-manifested solution. Don't get me wrong; what comes out of our mouths is extremely important. It is something we should be focused on and mindful of at all times. However, just because we change our words doesn't mean we have changed our hearts! "Faith comes by hearing, and hearing by the word,"[3] so it is vital to speak faith into our words and to get our hope stirred up from the inside, out—with the words that we're not only speaking, but are inevitably hearing!

What we believe, and knowing what we believe are vital to living a healthy, *wellthy* life. It will be apparent in the words we speak and the questions we ask. Beware: to simply focus on changing our words without taking a serious look at where those words are coming from would be as crazy as just giving someone a pill to stop a symptom. Why? To merely cover up a symptom while the devastating cause of that symptom is left undiscovered and undetermined can eventually lead to death!

In fact, I wonder how many heart attacks have occurred because someone was trying desperately to change their words and speak life, while all along an issue of the heart had never been dealt with. The longer I live, the more I realize how very little the degree of separation is between the spiritual and physical aspects of who I am, and who we are as people.

The more I study and see what is happening to people as they suffer from the serious disease of "dis-ease," the more I understand the importance of addressing life from the inside, out—and living it that way!

"God doesn't provide the solution, He is the solution!"

Earlier I mentioned the statement, "We talk about the problem while we believe God provides the solution." Interestingly, while I was writing that statement I realized, "God doesn't provide the solution, He *is* the solution!" Wow, now that's an interesting thought, isn't it?

If God is the solution, then we can seek Him as the solution; we can seek His face, not His hand. It's not what He can give us that makes us *wellthy*, but it is He who is *wellth*. And He has already made us *wellthy*.

When He is living on the inside of us, then within us lies the solution to every problem that we encounter, all because He is in us!

Here's the key: Live in Him. When you do, you are living in the solution! Your life is no longer your own, but "ours"; you plus God. That is the coolest thing ever! When you really understand what I just said, you will no longer speak the problem, because you will allow yourself to hear and listen to the solution by the very words coming out of your mouth, out of the abundance of your heart!

So what's it going to be? Are you going to speak life or are you going to speak death over your life? It's your choice. Are you going to take the next step or not? You get to decide.

The dictionary defines "decide" as "1. to arrive at a solution that ends uncertainty or dispute about 2. to bring to a definitive end 3. to induce, to come to a choice 4. to make a choice or judgment."[4] It comes from the Latin word *decidere*, which literally means "to cut off." When you decide, you cut off any other option, except of course, the ability to make another decision. Mediocrity is no longer an option. Failure is no longer an option. Sickness is no longer an option. Obesity or being overweight is no longer an option. Suffering is definitely not an option.

Now is your time to decide what you want to see manifested in your life. More health? More *wellth*? More life? More wealth? Some of the most powerful, infinitely creative words you can speak are the ones that manifest themselves in the questions you ask. Your life will be a result of the questions you ask, and the health and *wellth* of your life will be determined by how question-able you are. Asking great questions more often will lead to more great questions being asked of you. When you have the answers to the questions you are being asked, or you have the solutions to the problems you or others are having, your life becomes the answer and you will be both *wellthy* and wealthy!

I cannot write a book about how to be healthy and *wellthy* without sharing the truth with you about the source of all health, *wellth*, life, and wealth. It is God Himself. The most important question you will ever ask, and the one that will make you most question-able is this: "God, will you please save me?" To save you not only from the unthinkable eternity of hell, but just as important, from the hell you've been living in here on earth. You can do this by asking God's son, Jesus, to become the Lord of your life so you no longer have to do this life-thing alone. Jesus died on the cross for you. He became your sin and went to hell on your behalf so you would never have to. And then, He did the greatest thing of all—He conquered death by coming back to life so you and I could live an abundant, healthy, *wellthy* life! If that doesn't settle it once and for all, then nothing will.

When we ask Jesus into our hearts, it changes everything from the inside, out. He is our way to knowing God personally. He is in us and we are in Him. There is nothing we cannot do or cannot be. "With God all things are possible."[5] There is no need that He has not already fulfilled. We will have desires because He put those in us, but only to guide and direct us to fulfill the purpose that He has for us.

We no longer need to ask for anything, except wisdom and guidance. (And as many Afformations as we desire. ☺) He has already given us all we need for an abundant, Zoë-kind of life! This revelation has changed everything for me, including the way I pray. I used to pray and ask God for things. But if I already have eyes, why ask for eyes? If I already have ears, why ask for ears? Instead, I ask for eyes to see what He has already given me, and ears to hear instructions on putting every blessing to good use. I already have everything I need; I just ask that He allow me to receive it. You can, too!

A grateful life is a life full of great.

When I realized that God *is* the answer to my every prayer, all I could do was just thank Him and praise Him for who He is and what I am because of what Jesus did for me and you. Remember, a grateful life is a life full of great. And it's definitely a healthy, *wellthy* one!

As I said, I cannot write a book about how to experience health and *wellth* for life and not tell you the truth, even if it means that you may want to reject the rest of the information because somewhere, someone along your path has tried to shove this whole idea down your throat (in the name of some religion). The great news is, God is exactly *not* like that. He does not shove anything down our throats. God is not religion. In fact, He is the One who designed us with the ability to choose, also known as free will. I believe free will is essential to life, because once you attempt to take away someone's free will, you take away his or her power. Without power, the lights go out. Free will is *free* and my only question to you is: Are you willing to be free?

My sincere hope is that you will continue to be open to what I am saying to you. This message could literally save your life today!

God is the one who gives free will because God is love, and love is free, and love will set us free. Love is the greatest choice we have available to us. It is the most important cornerstone for building health and *wellth* for life. Otherwise, let's face it, if you don't have the power within you to take the actions necessary to live your best life, all you've got is some more good information, another great plan or program. But plans and programs don't guarantee great health and a healthy, *wellthy* life, and neither does eating well and exercise. In fact, Dr. Jim Richards, a man I respect very much, says this, "*Eating and exercise do not guarantee great health, but are merely a reflection of the great health and life that are already within you.*"

When you can reflect the power that is within you, the reflection is not only bold and bright, but it's lifesaving. It is somewhat like a lighthouse; it helps direct and save lives. The truth that I just shared with you is the same way. Its radiance will be seen in the life-giving words you speak and the life that you live as a result of those questions you dare to ask.

If you do not know God intimately, then I would like to help you do that. It's really quite simple. All you need to do is *ask*.

No one comes to know God without first being drawn to Him by His Spirit. Follow that desire in your heart as it comes and it will guide you into all truth and a knowing that goes deeper than words can explain. It is absolutely the most precious, powerful, profound, and entirely pure relationship I have ever had the privilege of having. God is real and so is His Son. I appreciate the opportunity to introduce you to them.

All you've got to do is ask, and you shall *receive*.

I am going to direct you to another book I wrote (*It's No Secret... When You Know the Truth, Your Steps Are Fulfilling*) that will help you immensely. You can go to www.drshannonknows.com and we will help you. All you need to do is ask!

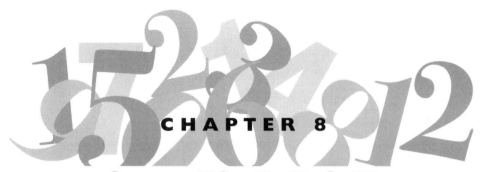

CHAPTER 8

Step #8: B.E.S.T. from A.D.I.O.

(Be Excellent Starting Today from Above Down Inside Out)

Did you know?

Your best leads to better...naturally.

Immense power stems from Being Excellent Starting Today, especially when it comes from Above, Down, Inside, and Out! (I love acronyms, can you tell? ☺) This is the health and *wellth* for life mind-set. It starts with fearlessly exposing yourself and asking, "Where am I?" Instead of comparing yourself to how you once were or to where you wish you were, you answer this question based on where you are today compared to God's best for you. Are you your best?

In the dictionary, "best" is defined as a superlative of good. "Good" is how God described you when He made you in His image. On the sixth day, He said, "and it was very good."[1] He made you good and that's that. Nothing you do can change that. The question is, are you being the best "very good" that you can be?

For fifteen to twenty years, there was a restaurant in Tulsa that absolutely made the best chicken. Many would define the chicken as being "something magical." In fact, if I described the legendary chicken to anyone within one hundred miles of here, they would know exactly which restaurant I was talking about.

The smoked chicken would literally fall off the bone with a flavor that commanded reactions like, "Whoa, that's unbelievable!" Although customers would eat until they could no longer fit any more in, the chicken would always keep them begging for more. The side dishes of fresh veggies, tabouli, and hummus completed the flavor perfection.

What was it about that place? Actually, the place itself was nothing special at all. It was a little hole-in-the-wall not far from my previous office. Yet, it was a clean place—as clean as filthy can be! The carpet was so old that only God Himself could imagine the stories that lay in the grit and grime of the age-old memories of past lunches and dinners. Most customers came in only to take their luscious chicken and healthy side dishes to go. Besides the food, there was nothing else good about it. Some say that the mysterious owner and his wife lived in the back of the restaurant. About this rumor, I am not quite sure.

What I am sure of is that there was always a line at the counter. The dingy bare walls displayed a few homemade signs such as: "No Substitutions Allowed. Period!"; "This is not a fast-food restaurant, but a slow-food restaurant"; and, "We reserve the right to refuse service to anybody."

The owner was what some would call "a friendly guy, but not!" Some likened him to the Soup Nazi from *Seinfeld*. I'm absolutely sure he told a customer or two over the years, "No chicken for you!" ☺ Furthermore, he did not answer the phone. And if he ran out of chicken, he would lock the doors for the day. Most never dared to ask him about his ingredients or which kind of oil he used to cook the chicken. He never accepted anything but the highest quality ingredients, so when a local crop shortage of tomatoes occurred, he temporarily stopped using them even though they were a crucial ingredient in his famous tabouli recipe. Even he did not make any substitutions. Being the generous man that he was, he wouldn't even think of increasing his prices to offset the effects of supply and demand!

Many local papers reviewed the restaurant and their articles were posted on the walls: five stars for food, two stars for service, and one star for atmosphere. Nonetheless, the restaurant was known as a legendary barbecue chicken place for years! Then the unthinkable happened.

One day, the owner just closed the doors and shut the restaurant down. The rumor was that he had some personal and family issues, so he moved back to the Middle East. Interestingly enough, many people attempted to buy his restaurant and the secret recipes for his famous chicken. But he refused! He was so proud of his product that he wasn't going to sell it to anyone, for any price. Instead, he just closed the doors and left the country, never sharing his secrets with anyone and leaving behind the luscious memories of the incredible chicken that many since have unsuccessfully attempted to duplicate.

By the way, I personally never ate his chicken, but have heard wonderful stories from several people who did. I'm married to one of them, and he is sure he knows the secret ingredient to the famous chicken because he knew the owner very well. That's a whole other story. ☺

Not long ago, a reputable restaurant owner in town opened a restaurant with a similar name and concept. Although it appears that he has replicated the product (but not quite; there still seems to be something missing), it still lacks that indefinable magic that cannot be overlooked even with the new space, fresh décor, and friendly service.

That missing "certain something" that is both indefinable and exquisite is known as greatness. It keeps everyone intrigued and magnetically attracted to its magnificence, causing moments of "Whoa," "Wow," and "Aha!" Greatness is what keeps us coming back for more.

A seed of greatness is excellence in its rawest form. The difference is, when you discover that excellence inside of you, you do not have to be excellent at everything; yet, you will be excellent in all. When you discover your best, the rest is easy.

Over the hill

One day God gave me a revelation on this concept of best. It was the same day that He specifically clarified my mission as a messenger of hope. He showed me that my mission is to work with people who want to become better by helping them to be their best. I was so excited!

As I've increased in years (my refusal to say, "*as I've gotten older*" must mean that I'm actually getting older ☺), I have wondered, "Does growing older mean I will always compare myself to how I used to be in the so-called 'good old days' when I was younger, stronger, blah, blah, blah?" I've always been bothered when I hear people talk about the past as if it was the greatest thing ever, because then I wonder, "Does that mean life can never be great again? Will life be all downhill from here, because compared to how it used to be, it's just not the same?" Then, I've thought about what a drag being sixty, seventy, eighty-plus years will be if it just means that the further we get from "the good old days" the less "good" our life will be! I think you get the picture.

Do you believe that? I refuse to believe that! Best is the opposite of the mind-set I just described. Best isn't about being twenty, thirty, sixty, or seventy; it's about being *fully alive today*! Living your best is "giving out of what you have, instead of refusing to give because you think you have not."

Your best is about giving and receiving with all you have and then some. Your best is about taking from the past and giving it all first, instead of saving it for last; it's about your very best until the very last! Your best is about coming from where you are right now and putting one foot forward—your best foot forward—and loving yourself regardless of where you were yesterday or where you are going tomorrow.

Best is not about becoming; best is about *being*. I love best because it's something you can always have on the inside of you, so it's something you can always be. I love best because it's like your tithe. God says we should give our best; our firstfruits, a tenth right off of the top—the cream of the crop.

Okay, maybe He didn't say those exact words. I guess you could call that Shannon's translation, but nonetheless, He wants our best. Some may say, "What if I don't have enough to give? He wants me to give 10 percent, but what if I can't afford that?" God never asked for ten dollars because some may not be able to afford ten dollars; instead, God asked for 10 percent of what you already have. If you have life flowing through you then you have something to give, even if that something is hope for a better tomorrow! This is exactly how best works!

God didn't ask for "better than." In fact, He doesn't like us to compare ourselves to others. Actually, I believe He doesn't even want us to compare our right hands to our left hands. God wants us to be who we are today; right here, right now. That's exciting, isn't it?

The djembe factor

Ever since I was ten years old, I have played the drums and been fascinated with rhythm. About ten years ago while visiting a friend in Syracuse, New York, I was introduced to hand drums when I bought my first djembe. (A djembe, pronounced jem-bay, is a West African drum that looks like a large goblet—round on top, tapering to a small hole on the bottom. You can play it with your hands while holding it between your knees so the sound can resonate out of the bottom, or you can put it on a stand and play it, like I do.)

Years ago my pastor asked if I would play my djembe in the praise and worship band at church. After prayerful consideration, I very enthusiastically agreed and have been having a blast ever since! The only thing better than playing the djembe for fun is playing it for the Lord!

One Sunday I was out of town and unable to participate in praise and worship at church. I realized that although I love the part I play in our service, the band continues playing just fine without me. Our lead drummer, on the other hand, would be sorely missed if he were gone. In fact, without our drummer, it would change everything because he is the backbone of the entire band. I, however, just add to what the drummer and bass player are doing. My contribution is that of bringing that little extra something. Can the band do without the djembe or other percussion instruments? Absolutely. But oh, it is so much more fun and flavorful with them!

It was then that I decided how important it is to bring fun and flavor to the functionality of life; to bring extra to the ordinary and praise to the worship. I call this the djembe factor.

Is your life lacking that extra zest, zeal, or zany rhythm that only you can bring?

Is your life lacking that extra zest, zeal, or zany rhythm that only you can bring? How's your djembe factor? Are you playing the best you can in the song of your life?

Once again, are you being your best today? That is the question or maybe that is the answer to the question, "Where are you?" It's all about where you are in relation to who you are, and whether or not you are being that "who" today. If your answer isn't exciting to you because you can't say "Yes, I am my best right now!" then it's time to check your heart. Your best is more about your heart than your head, more about your heart than your circumstances. *Even if you're at your lowest point, you need to ask yourself, "What is my best right now? What does that look like?"*

Best to better

On some days, just being honest enough to truthfully and wholeheartedly answer this question regardless of what you think you should say is your best. Being your best is about being real and honest (real honest). Where are you today and who are you being? Your best is about your willingness to accept where you are today. No excuses, no condemnation, and no shame!

Acceptance is not the same as condoning. Acceptance is about awareness. Most people think better needs to come before best, when in essence best leads to better.

It's time to join the revolution! I believe that "health and *wellth* for life" is a mind-set, and it's the best mind-set. Unfortunately, the mind-set of the majority of people, especially those in America, is a mind-set of unhealthiness, sickness, dysfunction, poverty, "*less than*" or "*not enough.*" I believe this is one of the reasons we are suffering from what I call the "supersize me" epidemic. So many Americans believe they are not enough, which leads them to excess in all areas of their lives. I've got news for you: *you are more than enough!* And the best news is that you are more than enough *just the way you are!* If you can grab hold of this mind-set, excess and "supersize" will no longer seem necessary. You will no longer be needy or greedy, or feel the need to be greedy. Are you thinking, "*Me,* greedy?" If today you are robbing from your future, then you're greedy! Surprised?

Please do not feel condemned; all of us have suffered from this in some degree or another, including me.

If we don't stop the insanity, bigger will never be enough; and the truth is, life will become shorter. It's true! A 2010 *TIME* article stated, "…experts fear that this generation of American kids may be the first ever to have a shorter life span than their parents."[2] This is completely outrageous and unacceptable! It is time we say, "Enough is enough!" It is time we take our stand! It is time you take *your* stand and say, "No more!"

It's time to look at life from a different perspective; the best perspective. The best perspective is one from Above, Down, Inside, and Out. When you stand on the ground and look up on a cloudy day, you cannot see the sun. But does that mean the sun isn't shining?

When she was real little, I remember asking my daughter, "Anni, is the sun shining today?" She quickly responded, "The sun is always shining, Mama. It's just that we can't always see it." Then she smiled, as I almost choked back tears of amazement. How did she get so smart? ☺

We live in a culture that tells us health comes from the outside in, and if we are not feeling healthy, we must add something in from the outside. If that doesn't work, then we need to add more; then if that doesn't work, we need to start taking parts out until we do feel better. This simply is not true! Pills are not the answer to your pain; and again, pain is not your problem. Actually, the source of your pain is your problem. And until you deal with the cause of that pain, instead of just continuing to cover it up with drugs, your problem is not going to go away!

Every day people are dying at the hands of medicine. "Death By Medicine," a very comprehensive report written in November 2003 by Gary Null, PhD, Carolyn Dean, MD, ND, Martin Feldman, MD, Debora Rasio, MD, and Dorothy Smith, PhD, showed overwhelming evidence "that the American medical system is the leading cause of death and injury in the United States."[3] Based on the most conservative figures and statistics available in 2003, these doctors projected the occurrence of an estimated 7,841,360 deaths due to medical intervention over a ten-year span.[4] Given the fact that this report was written in the year 2003, the ten-year mark will be the year 2013. The report also states that "7.8 million iatrogenic deaths is more than all the casualties from all the wars fought by the US throughout its entire history."[5] *Today* is the day for you to live your best life—not yesterday, not tomorrow. Do not wait until your health is gone before you start becoming better by being your best.

Basking in *wellth*

Like the sun, your health and *wellth* are a shining source of life. Are you experiencing health and *wellth,* or are they trying to shine through the clouds of bad perspective and bad principle? It is vital for you to tap into your health and to intimately *know* your *wellth* to truly be the healthy, *wellthy* person you were designed and destined to be! You see, when you know your innate value, you will cherish the *wellth* and health that's within you. You will live from *within*, instead of from *without.* I truly believe that you must experience something to be something, so once you know your *wellth* and experience it, you will be both *wellthy* and healthy! *Wellth* is the source of your health. When you know your *wellth*, you will prosper in health.

Are you expressing your best? Your best health? Your best *wellth*?

Have you ever wondered what your best life would look like? Accordingly, have you ever wondered what "best" really means? I'd love to tell you! "Best" is a superlative of "good" and means "1. of a favorable character or tendency 2. BOUNTIFUL, FERTILE 3. ...ATTRACTIVE 4. SUITABLE, FIT 5. SOUND, WHOLE 6. AGREEABLE, PLEASANT 7. ...WHOLESOME 8. CONSIDERABLE, AMPLE 9. FULL 10. WELL-ROUNDED 11.TRUE 12. legally valid or effectual 13. ADEQUATE, SATISFACTORY...COMMENDABLE, VIRTUOUS, KIND."[6]

Did you know that another word for "best" is "well"? Words such as: "to rise up and flow out, in a good or proper manner: RIGHTLY, EXCELLENTLY, SKILLFULLY, SATISFACTORILY, FORTUNATELY, ABUNDANTLY, COMPLETELY, FULLY, PROSPEROUS and HEALTHY, or free or recovered from ill health"[7] are used to define the word "well." Isn't that awesome?

Isn't this the most incredible definition? Did you know that best actually meant all those wonderful things? And what's with "prosperous" in the middle of that definition? Did you know that prosperity isn't just about money, but it's about best? Prosperity is about being very good— being well! It's about being *wellthy*!

Hand in hand

I guess you can see why I talk about health and *wellth* together. You can't have one without the other. True prosperity is about being your best. It's been my experience that when we are being our best, financial prosperity and abundance also come. I don't know about you, but that's intriguing to me. So many people go after financial gain and material riches first and in the process become so much less than their best. The key to incredible wealth (*wellth*, as I like to call it) is to be your best. All else will follow naturally.

The best way to be your best is to work with what you already have.

The best way—yes, I believe it is the best way—to be your best is to work with what you already have. To do this, give from what you already have. So often, we think that in order to be our best we need to add to ourselves; add to our finances, add to our bodies (don't even get me started on this one!). The best way to live is to care for the resources we already have on the inside of us and on the outside of us in the place we call home.

This whole idea of outside-in thinking has caused so much destruction on our planet. Life begins on the inside and continues from the inside, out. All life flows from above, down, inside, and out from your brain, to your body, to your life! This is how life flows, and it's exactly how health and healing occur.

Nothing happens in your body without your brain. Everything works because the brain tells it to work. (Yes, that's right!) The principle of Above, Down, Inside, and Out is going to do more for your health for life than you realize.

The nervous system is the most powerful force available to us besides the power of God. Actually I believe the nervous system is the very power of God flowing through us. The power that made the body is the power that heals the body. As long as there is no interference to this power flowing through us, we are healthy and function properly. If there is interference, it's like you have a kink in the garden hose that waters your favorite garden; the garden will not flourish. The flowers may live, but are they *fully* alive? As the flowers struggle to flourish, weeds start to grow in even the most unlikely soil. This is exactly how disease happens.

So many people think that disease comes from germs, when in reality, disease occurs when the host ("the soil") is ripe for germs to germinate and grow. If the soil is well-nurtured and nutrient-rich, there will be no room for germs or weeds to take root. This is why you can be working in an office full of people and only a few people "catch" the cold that is going around. But I ask you, did the cold catch them or did they catch it? Have you ever noticed that it always seems to be the same people who "catch" whatever seems to be floating around? Is it the individuals who are genuinely happy, eating well, exercising, and speaking life? Or is it the Debbie-Downers who drink soda, eat donuts, smoke, and are always complaining? Now I'm not saying that people who eat well and exercise will never become s-i-c-k. (I don't like to say or even write that four-letter word, so I spelled the letters out individually here instead.) I believe there is immense power in the words we speak, so before you say this word, especially after the two very powerful words "I am," you had better be aware of what you are saying.

Do not claim to be something you do not choose to be!

You may be asking yourself, "What does she mean by all of this? What should I say when I feel less than optimal?" Well, you can try saying what I say: "I feel less than optimal (aka "L.T.O.") or "I feel symptomatic, but I am overcoming."

When I have felt L.T.O., it's usually been after I haven't nurtured my soil; I've allowed it to run low on nutrients, low on sunshine, low on rest, etc. When I feel less than optimal, my immediate checklist is: (1) am I getting my nervous system checked and adjusted on a regular basis? (2) am I eating well? (3) am I eating too much sugar? (4) am I drinking enough water? (5) am I resting well? (6) am I exercising regularly? and (7) how is my stress level?

Usually, one or more of these areas is drastically out of balance. Once I identify it, I do my best to correct it. Remember, symptoms such as pain are not the problem; the cause of the pain or other symptoms is the problem. Pain doesn't kill people, but the problem can. Therefore, why would you want to cover up pain when its purpose is to warn you of danger? That would be as absurd as unplugging the red light when it comes on in a vehicle or pounding on the dashboard in the hopes that the problem will go away. It may be time to look under the hood or at the frame.

So my question to you is this, "Who is your chiropractor?" If your answer is, "I don't have a chiropractor," then that is the first place to start. Find one. Are you thinking, "Why is chiropractic such a big deal?"

Chiropractors help locate and correct the cause of less-than-optimal health. They do not merely cover up symptoms with drugs! *I'm not telling you this because I am a chiropractor. To the contrary, I am a chiropractor because I believe this philosophy and live by the principles I am teaching you because of what I am about to share with you.* I hope you get a hold of what I'm about to tell you because it has the power to not only help you experience health and *wellth* for life, but it has the potential to save your life and the lives of those you love.

Innate Intelligence is the vital force of life within your body.

Did you know there is something in every living thing that keeps it alive? Well, I know; and if you do not, you're about to. It's true—it's in you and it's in me! It's called "Innate Intelligence" and I believe God put it there. Some people call it the electricity or the power of the body. For example, right now your heart is beating, but do you know why it's beating? Because your body's Innate Intelligence is telling it to beat. It's the vital force of life within your body! It's been there since you were conceived. An egg and a sperm came together and began to divide…and finally your brain and spinal cord, the lifeline of your body, were formed.

Our brain sits up in our skull. There is a hole in the bottom of the skull called the foramen magnum. There is also a hole in the first bone of the spine called the atlas vertebrae, as well as in every vertebra of the spine. The brain stem, which is an extension of the brain, branches through the spine as the spinal cord. Your spinal cord is the *brain* in your back. Your nervous system and life flow through the body from Above, Down, Inside, and Out. Are you beginning to see how important your nervous system is, as well as the spine that surrounds it?

Innate Intelligence is fully capable of running all the functions that constitute life, which are growth, replacement of worn-out tissues, and repair of fracture and other injuries. It's responsible for your body's incredible innate self-healing ability!

I don't think many people would argue that it requires intelligence to build the body *and* keep it alive. Your central nervous system is the intelligent master control system and the lifeline to your whole body.

Hopefully, you are beginning to see that chiropractic is not just about aches and pains. Symptoms are simply warning signs, just like that red light coming on in your car. Chiropractic is about optimal health and *wellth* from Above, Down, Inside, and Out.

Interference to the nervous system results in a loss of optimal health (and *wellth*). Your lifeline is protected by bone, which is the skull and spinal column. The trillions of nerve fibers that flow through the atlas region out to the rest of the body control every organ and cell in the body! Did you know that? It's amazing, isn't it?

Vertebral subluxations (spinal misalignments) cause interference to the flow of life from Above, Down, Inside, and Out. What was designed to protect the nervous-system function (your spinal column) also has the ability to interfere with its proper function. It is absolutely vital to discover the cause of any dysfunction in your body versus merely covering up or masking the symptoms.

My experience is that dysfunction in the body is caused by interference to the nervous system (or lifeline of your body). Specific, scientific chiropractic adjustments slowly and gradually remove interference to the proper function of the nervous system. This takes both time and repetition, not unlike building your body. You don't get into the best shape of your life by working out only once in a while, or the first time you jump on a treadmill or lift a weight at the gym. It even takes nine months for a new life to form and be born, so why would we think that healing should happen overnight? Much the same, disease does not occur overnight. Sometimes it can take years to manifest, and symptoms are usually the last thing to show up.

Time and repetition are two components of the healing process that I don't personally enjoy, but healing is all about consistency. Consistent bodily functions such as respiration and a beating heart make the most impact in your life. Try this: Take a deep breath in, and then let it out. How simple was that? *But oh so vital! Health* and *wellth* are about life flowing through you daily and consistently at 100 percent. What is essential for your life is absolutely essential for your health and *wellth*.

> ## "Rome wasn't built in a day, symptoms don't arise in a day, and healing doesn't happen in a day."

"Rome wasn't built in a day, symptoms don't arise in a day, and healing doesn't happen in a day" (Dr. Schiffman). Your life isn't just one day…but it's about living it one day at a time, the best way you can. It's time to make "healthy" your new habit!

What you don't know, won't hurt you?

In the early stages of *vertebral subluxation*, there are no symptoms. Imagine that! It's no different than the fact that tooth cavities don't start out as toothaches—sometimes it can take years to feel the pain of decay! However, if you are having any pain in your back, neck, head, or teeth, there is a good chance that the cause of your symptoms has been there for a long, long, long time!

You may be wondering what causes *vertebral subluxations* (spinal misalignments). Life can cause them because we are designed with lots of moveable parts. Trauma, falls, accidents, emotions, toxins, stress, and the birthing process are just a few of the many causes of subluxation.

I remember holding a baby for the first time when I was a kid. My mom told me to support the back's neck and not to touch the "soft spot" on top of the baby's head. As delicate as their heads and necks are, the birthing process can be very traumatic for both the newborn and the mom. I'm not sure if you have ever seen a pair of forceps, but they basically look like big metal salad tongs. These tongs are placed around the baby's head and neck and the baby is pulled out! At times, babies are vacuum extracted out of their mothers. The suction cup is placed on their delicate skulls and they are virtually sucked out! Wow! Sometimes people think that delivering a baby via C-section is the way to go, and less traumatic for the baby. Unfortunately, these babies are still pulled out of their mothers' wombs by their heads and necks. Ironically, the first thing we're told when we hold a baby is to be careful how we hold the newborn's head and neck!

Are you starting to see why every newborn should be evaluated for *vertebral subluxations* as soon as possible after birth? It is absolutely vital!

Over the years I have seen a great many babies, children, and adults who have suffered with such things as colic, ear infections, reflux, constipation, sinus problems, allergies, menstrual problems, depression, headaches, migraines, neck pain, upper back pain, lower back pain, shoulder pain, knee pain, leg pain, foot pain, and more. I have also had the joy of watching countless numbers of people heal from such things!

Is it because I am a miracle worker? No. It is because I get to work with the miracle of life every time I lay my hands on someone. There is no greater joy than seeing someone get better because they are committed to being their best!

The more you understand the power of your nervous system, and the importance of its functioning with no interference, the healthier and *wellthier* you will be. Living this way is about so much more than symptoms or no symptoms; it's about living with "full expression of life" (my personal definition of health).

So what does all of this have to do with being your best? I believe with all my heart that it is impossible to be your best without fully expressing yourself from Above, Down: From God to you, from your head to your heart, from your brain to your body, and from your head to your toe. And from the Inside, Out: From you to the world, from your heart to humanity, from the center to the periphery, and from within to "no longer without"!

Another way to understand this Above, Down, Inside, Out principle is to think of it this way: The power that makes the body is the power that heals the body. Being our best is about addressing all that comes our way from the resources we have on the inside, versus substituting something from the outside, in.

The central nervous system was the first organ to form, and out of that came everything else. It is "the center" for a reason, and if we don't address it in all situations, we are in danger because we miss its power that leads to life in the first place. And life is essential for healing, health, and *wellth*!

At your best, or just like the rest?

If you are going to be your best, you must define or redefine your personal definition of health (and *wellth*) and it must include the defining function of the power that created you in the first place. The A.D.I.O.

principle is what separates you from all of your symptoms and circumstances. I find it quite intriguing that *a dio* means "to God" in Italian. Perhaps the principle of Above, Down, Inside, Out helps reconnect our physical bodies to the God who designed them in the first place.

So now how do *you* define health (and *wellth*)? And is your health defining you at your best or just like the rest?

Perhaps it's time for you to take the next step.

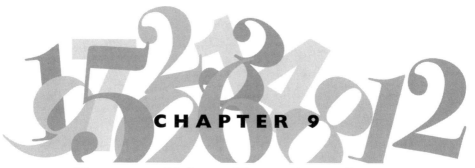

CHAPTER 9

Step #9: Be 1 of 11

Did you know?

*The only thing more powerful than a vision
is the power of a shared vision.*

"So, who keeps you straight?"

That's exactly what my dear friend Michael asked me one day. He's great at posing wonderful, thought-provoking questions. This particular question held the beginning of an answer that has manifested itself in many new and amazing relationships, including meeting the man of my dreams—my dear husband, the best partner a girl could ever ask for. ☺ (By the way, I also have a great chiropractor who *keeps me straight.*)

Who keeps me straight?

The questions others ask us are not nearly as powerful as those we ask ourselves. So I encourage you to ask yourself, Who keeps me straight? Who's going to help me reach my goals, dreams, and desires? Who is going to help me be healthy and *wellthy*?

The importance of having someone or someone(s) in your life to help keep you on track and hold you accountable is significant. So, what does "accountable" mean anyway? *Answerable.*[1] Seriously! You can have the greatest vision imaginable and a proven, effective plan or program; but without a strategy that includes trustworthy, answerable accountability, it's almost impossible to succeed. So how do you go about selecting your partner?

Without Step #4 (Be Answerable) and Step #7 (Be Question-able), Step #9 is very difficult. In fact, I believe it's almost impossible. Why? Unless you have taken responsibility for where you are and can ask for help, you will not be able to choose the right partner. I've got news for you; you cannot live a healthy, *wellthy* life alone! You need others to help you. We all do, and others need you and me as well.

First, ask yourself, "What do I desire? What is my vision?" Second, ask God to help you. Third, ask that special someone to join with you in accomplishing your mission. Perhaps someone has already been asking you to join their cause. It's possible that your partner(s) has been there all along, but you just haven't recognized him or her, or you haven't said yes, or dared to ask. It may be as simple as asking someone to train with you or be your trainer.

> *One can do so much,*
>
> *but two can do so much more!*

One can do so much, but two can do so much more! That is the power of relationship; the right relationship. With the right relationship and the exponential power of agreement, the results have the potential to positively affect multitudes.

The Power of 1 and 1

Anyone who knows me knows that my favorite number is eleven. What I like most about the number eleven is that it's two #1s side by side. Who wouldn't want a double helping of #1? Twice the fun, twice the victory, twice the strength, twice the collaboration, twice the celebration! You see, 1 and 1 isn't 2, it's 11!

There is infinite power when two come together, especially in agreement. One can do so much, but two can do so much more. As you know, God designed some birds to instinctually fly south for the winter. Imagine what would happen to a bird if it attempted to head out on its own. I imagine a painfully difficult and, I believe, impossible journey! (And "impossible" isn't a word I like to use!)

So often we go through life trying to do it on our own, trying to make our own way, when all along other people, (other "ones") are there to help us. I call them divine connections. Why? Because there is nothing more divine than a true connection!

We were never meant to do life alone. We're programmed to believe that we need to look out for "number one." But what if you go through life and have 100 percent of very little, when you could have had 50 percent of a whole lot! When you share what you have, it multiplies exponentially. Eventually, when you partner together, you end up with 100 percent of a whole lot. *Everyone wins!*

Partnering is not even about giving and taking; it's about sharing and receiving. When we begin to focus on what we can share, instead of on what we can receive, what we have to share *grows*. When we begin to focus on what we have, instead of what we have not, what we have *grows*. More importantly, who we are *grows* exponentially. The end result is even more to share. It's awesome!

Accountability is absolutely vital to our success, and more importantly, whether or not we will even make the journey. A written goal is so much more likely to be realized than an unwritten one, but a goal written and shared is achieved and multiplied by 1 and 1. I don't know about you, but I want to be a goal achiever, not just a goal setter. Do you agree?

Being your best isn't just about you; it's about everyone else being their best because they are sharing this ride with you. If you don't share the greatness that's on the inside of you, then someone else is not going to be able to receive it, and therefore, they will have less to share with others. We all need each other to be our best.

The problem is, most people think they need to be more in order to give more, so they don't give at all. The truth is, unless we share what we have, we won't have more to share.

Am I making any sense to you? Sharing is not an "if, then" but an "I, when" experience. You will be all that you *can be*, when you realize that you *already are* more than enough, and celebrate what and who you are! Do yourself a favor; read that again slowly.

Are you expressing your greatness? Are you sharing your "oneness" (your uniqueness) with other "ones"? Are you waiting for your partner to give 50 percent before you give 50 percent? Two halves don't make a whole—one and one wholes do. How about giving 100 percent so that no matter what anyone else gives in your life, your experience is 100 percent full and fulfilling!

How about celebrating your life and those in it, because what you celebrate will *grow*. (Remember Step #5.) Again, 1 and 1 really does equal 11!

Do you believe in yourself?

health4life REVOLUTION!

So who's the "one" who is going to help you succeed? The right partner, coach, mentor, friend is someone who believes in you. We all need someone to believe in us, and we especially need to believe in ourselves. Success starts here: Do you believe in yourself? If so, what are you willing to do with that belief?

Even the best athletes in the world have a coach, and many of them have a chiropractor. I've learned some of the greatest lessons in my life from my coaches and chiropractors, and they have helped me be who I am today. If you are looking for a health coach (aka chiropractor), you can check out my Web site at www.drshannonknows.com.

Since 2001, I have been teaching a specific eating and exercise plan to help successfully transform individuals, corporations, and communities. Within as little as four weeks, people begin to see noticeable changes in their health and *wellth*. Within as little as four hours per week, people's lives begin to change. In twelve weeks, the transformations are incredible. Log on, and see for yourself!

The next two chapters outline this plan, the *health4life REVOLU-TION!* but let me first remind you of Step #4 (Be Answerable), because *you* are the one responsible for your decision to take the next step. You are responsible for any and all risks and results that could be associated with beginning an eating and exercise program. Please consult a medical or health professional before you start, especially if you have any questions about your health or ability to follow the eating and exercise plan contained in the following two chapters. The best advice I can give you is to weigh your risks and ask yourself, "Is it riskier or potentially hazardous to my health to do absolutely nothing?" I urge you to take responsibility, get questions to your answers, and be the answer to your questions!

Now, are you ready to become part of the *health4life REVOLUTION!* and join the movement?

CAUTION:

CONSULT YOUR PHYSICIAN BEFORE MAKING

SIGNIFICANT CHANGES IN NUTRITIONAL HABITS

OR BEGINNING NEW FORMS OF EXERCISE.

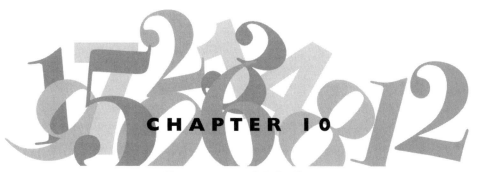

CHAPTER 10

Step #10:
Eat Responsibly for Life!

Did you know?

Your body is a temple and littering is strictly prohibited.
— a Jamba Juice napkin quote

Are you hungry for the truth?

One day I was driving behind a white minivan and noticed a rear-window decal that said "Eat Responsibly." So often, we pay no attention to what goes into our mouths! Thomas Moffett says, "We are digging our graves with our teeth." We have been blessed with a wonder-filled, magnificent body that deserves to be well fed and cared for. It's a large responsibility.

Are you ready to be responsible? Perhaps I should rephrase that and say, "Are you ready and willing to be answerable?" (Step #4 Be Answerable).

Are you ready to eat responsibly *for life*? Are you ready to *shop* responsibly *for life*?

If you want to eat better, you must shop better!

If you want to eat better, you must shop better! We often think we can buy whatever junk food we desire, telling ourselves we'll have the willpower to not eat it when we get home. (By the way, just some "food for thought": There is really no such thing as "junk food." It's either junk or it's food!) Do you really think that if you come home hungry in a very stressed-out mood, you will eat only one piece of chocolate? From my experience, chocolate was never meant to be eaten that way! I don't know about you, but if I buy a bag of chocolates, each piece cries out to me every time I walk through my kitchen. ☺

My rule with chocolate or ice cream is this: *Go out for it!* Buy it, eat it, enjoy it, and *do not* return to your house with it. That way it's a purposeful pleasure, instead of a future regret. If you don't want it in the temple, don't bring it into your home!

Out of all the topics I've spoken about over the years, nutrition seems to draw the biggest crowd. It gets the most attention, and at the same time, the least in attention to action. Could it be that "interest alone" equals "ignorance"? People, especially Americans, don't do what they know (or *think* they know) to do when it comes to eating well. In fact, I'm shocked at how ignorant most people really are when it comes to healthful eating and proper nutrition.

Everyone seems to be looking for a quick fix, the magic formula, the secret to weight loss. That search has driven people in this country to spend billions each year! According to the "Global Weight Management Report" by Markets and Markets, "The global weight management market is estimated to reach US$586 billion in 2014 from about US$365 billion in 2009,"[1] yet we are still fatter and unhealthier than ever.

> ## "There is no diet, or drug for that matter, that leads to health for life."

Why is that? There are as many diets out there as we are willing to buy into, but please hear me when I say, "There is no diet, or drug for that matter, that leads to health for life." Diets simply do not work! If they did, we would be a thin, fit, healthy people.

Is your food controlling you?

For years, I've taught the *health4life REVOLUTION! program*—which encompasses the *E.A.T.4life plan*, described in this chapter, and *H.i.T.4life plan* (in the next chapter)—to groups around the nation. In so doing, I've watched people attain incredible results; life-changing transformations, to say the least. Many times, the people who come to me proclaiming they've tried everything but can't lose weight are the people who experience the greatest results. I believe it's because what I teach them is how to live their best lives and when they do, their bodies function at their best—naturally!

My desire is for you to have a healthy relationship with food; to eat based on how you choose to care for your body, to eat what you desire when you choose to eat it, and to do so with power and freedom. It's time to exercise your power to choose what, when, and why you eat. This is your time to stop being controlled by food, whether you're fat or fit.

What do I mean by that? I see many overweight people who are controlled by food, but I also see just as many fit people who are equally controlled by food. These fit people are seemingly in control of what they eat, but they're ruled by their obsession of how they eat or don't eat, or how they exercise or don't exercise. Both types of people are not living in freedom. They're controlled by how they view food.

It's not so much what you eat, but what is eating you! *You* are what matters! Are you empowered when you eat, or are you entangled in a mess of unhealthy thoughts and actions? Are you in control of yourself, or is your food controlling you?

If your answer is, "Yes, my food is controlling me," are you surprised at this discovery? And now that you're aware, what are you going to do with your "knowing"? Let's change your mind-set right here and now.

Who told you that you couldn't lose weight? Who told you that you need chocolate, caffeine, or sugar? Who told you that you're big-boned, so you've accepted a heavy body? Who told you that you're unable to reject fast food? Who told you that you are overweight because you're over forty? Who told you that you can't eat raw food and get the nutrients and tastiness you desire? *Who told you?*

It's time to set yourself free! It's time to tell yourself the truth. *Knowing* the truth is what sets you free. Without freedom, it is very difficult to experience health for life.

> *The power to choose is as simple as mind over matter, or perhaps* mind over fatter.

You *do* have the power to choose a different outcome. You have the power to choose a different way of shopping. You have the power to choose a different way of eating. You have the power to choose a new way of thinking. The power to choose is as simple as mind over matter, or perhaps mind over fatter. Condemnation and shame can lead to fat. Guilt can lead to fat. Control can lead to fat. Unforgiveness, especially toward oneself, can lead to fat. Fear can lead to fat. Imbalance in any area of your life and loss of peace can lead to fat.

Are you getting the picture? Perhaps it's time to lose the extra weights you've been carrying around—those loads that you and your aching back were never meant to carry. It's time you saw the truth.

What you need is not another weight-loss program. What you need is to see the truth, *know* the truth, and allow the truth to transform your mind; and then, the truth will radically transform your health and your life, from the inside, out. You will not need a *diet* when you learn how to *live it*.

Losing the diet mentality

You are where you are today because of how you've seen yourself—how you've thought about yourself and how you've felt about your body—the words you've spoken, and the actions you've taken (or have not taken). The great news is that you have the power to change your thoughts, feelings, words, actions, and health for a life beyond your wildest dreams!

Your choices will lead you to the results you desire, and instead of being a victim, you will rise up a victor (a champion!). This is so important! That is why Steps #1-#9 are foundational for what we are talking about here. If you don't settle these things once and for all, you will use the *E.A.T.4life* plan I'm going to give you as just another diet and it will not lead you to health or *wellth*.

In fact, when you live your life for a number on the scale, every time you step on it you may be programming yourself for weight gain. *How?* If every time you eat you find yourself thinking, "I hope I don't gain weight from this," or "If I eat this, I may gain weight," you may actually be causing yourself to gain weight because of all the fear, guilt, condemnation, and shame you are causing yourself. The scale can actually become your stumbling block. *You* are in control of your health and happiness, not your scale! Besides, I've heard that the subconscious mind doesn't recognize the word "don't." If this is true, can you imagine saying, "I hope I gain weight from this"? Yikes! Choose your thoughts and your words wisely.

My recommendation is this: If you desire to lose weight, do not weigh yourself more than once a week. When you weigh, use the same scale at the same time of day.

It's time to stop dieting and relying on the diet mentality, and to start living fully and healthfully for life. Your physical body is a representation of your thoughts. You may just be thinking too much. Excessive thinking on heavy, unhealthy thoughts, leads exactly to where we are as people— *fat, sick, and tired!*

Does this food feed the life I desire?

Are you getting this? It's time to be all you were created to be; no more, no less! It is time to eat for life. Ask yourself, "Does this food feed the life I desire, or not? Does this food feed the healthy body I desire, or not?"

The organic lifestyle

In 1997, I became a vegetarian, and for the first time in a very long time, my digestive system improved immensely. I no longer suffered from the stomach pain that I experienced almost every time I ate. In the past few years, I've added some meat back into my diet, but only on rare occasions.

I eat organic raw fruits and veggies as much as possible, and have learned much about the benefits of eating raw. What is "raw"? Raw means that your food has not been cooked over 105-118 degrees Fahrenheit. Raw is uncooked fruits, vegetables, seeds, and sprouted nuts and grains.

Raw is live food that is more nutritious and easily digestible.[2,3] More life in, means more life to live—that's my conclusion.

What is so fascinating is that raw is so much more than celery sticks and apples. There is an entire world of gourmet raw food out there! You would be amazed at how brilliant and creative these recipes are. I encourage you to check out some of the great raw-cuisine cookbooks and Web sites.

So, let's talk organic. Some people say it's better, some say it isn't. I say, organic is the best! I was raised on organic food from our family garden before organic food was the "in" or "cool" thing. It wasn't something my family called "organic"; we just called it "food." It wasn't until I was in college that I tasted "non-organic" fruits and vegetables, and I wondered why they tasted so different from the carrots or apples I ate from our garden—dirt and all! I don't absolutely love vegetables, so if I'm going to eat them, I want all the flavor and potential health benefit I can get! Don't you?

The dirty dozen

According to the Environmental Working Group, we can reduce our exposure to "pesticide residue"[4] by 80 percent[5] when we avoid the so-called "dirty dozen"[6]— the most contaminated fruits and vegetables. Here is the list, in order, starting with the worst:

1. Celery
2. Peaches
3. Strawberries
4. Apples
5. Blueberries
6. Nectarines
7. Bell Peppers
8. Spinach

9. Kale

10. Cherries

11. Potatoes

12. Grapes (imported)

Although it's always a good idea to rinse all produce, it doesn't eliminate pesticide exposure, especially for these particular fruits and vegetables. "The growing consensus among scientists is that small doses of pesticides and other chemicals can cause lasting damage to human health, especially during fetal development and early childhood."[7] Eating only five fruits and vegetables a day from this list, we consume ten pesticides on average![8] A CNN story on June 1, 2010, said, "If you're eating non-organic celery today, you may be ingesting sixty-seven pesticides with it, according to a new report from the Environmental Working Group."[9]

Shocking, huh? *So eat organic,* especially when it comes to the "dirty dozen"!

Shopping tips

First, do not go shopping when you're hungry. Instead, go after you've just finished a fabulous workout, have eaten a fulfilling meal, and are feeling as healthy as ever.

Second, shop at a local food co-op or a store that carries organic food, especially one that offers locally grown produce. That way, you'll buy healthful food and bless your community at the same time. Make sure you purchase organically grown produce, meat, eggs, etcetera, whenever you possibly can.

If our food isn't alive,

how do we expect it to keep us alive?

Third, stay on the perimeter of the grocery store as much as possible. Avoid the interior aisles as often as you can! The perimeter of the store is where you'll find the live, life-giving food, whereas the interior aisles contain boxes of manufactured, processed, dead food. If our food isn't alive, how do we expect it to keep us alive? Now, I'm not saying that you cannot purchase food from the aisles. I'm just saying that it's best to eat as little boxed or canned food as possible.

That leads me to the fourth tip: Choose raw food whenever possible; the more colorful, the better. My favorite is *green*. It really is time to *go green*! If you cannot get fresh fruits and produce, then frozen is the next best. Canned food is my least favorite. If you do choose food in a can, jar, or box, always (yes, I mean *always*) read the label! You'd be surprised at what manufacturers put into a box and call food. Pay special attention to labels that say "natural" and to box designs that look "healthy." The box may look healthy (you're not eating the box anyway!), but what's inside may not be. Natural doesn't always mean healthful, especially with all the added flavors, colors, and preservatives. If you cannot pronounce the name of the ingredient, do not put it in your body! And, just because a food item is organic and you purchased it at a health food store doesn't mean it's good for you.

I have a friend who buys organic cupcakes and muffins from a health food store, and thinking they're healthful, she eats several at a time. I used to eat in a similar way, until the day I realized that organic sugar is still sugar and organic oil is still fat! So don't be fooled!

Fifth, eat food in its most healthful, most whole, and whenever possible, most raw form. Let's face it, most of us don't love to eat vegetables (hopefully you do), so if we're going to eat them, we might as well get the maximum benefit from them. That's my rule of thumb, and it works for me. If you give it a chance, I believe it will work for you, too.

My sixth and final shopping tip is this: Use herbs liberally (cilantro, basil, dill, etcetera). They add so much incredible flavor to your food, as well as more nutrients.

The following eating strategy is a list of healthful foods for you to choose from. If you discover a healthful food that is not on the list, please let me know. I would love to add it to mine. Use this list to create an eating plan for yourself each day.

To help you, I have provided the following information in a free, easy-to-use list. You can request a copy on my Web site, www.drshannon-knows.com. This entire list is formatted on a very convenient and efficient 8 ½ x 11 inch sheet so you can have it at your fingertips when you plan and shop. The second sheet includes a place to write your goals so you have them in front of you at all times.

I suggest you print the sheets (front and back), laminate them, and use a dry erase marker to check off the items you need to pick up on your next shopping adventure. Remember, healthy shopping leads to healthy eating. I hope this sheet will help you immensely. Use it daily and weekly until this way of eating and living becomes second nature to you, and it will.

Even then, it's always wise to plan. It isn't that you have failed when it comes to eating, but that you have failed to plan. Anything worthwhile is worth your time, especially for your best life, your best health, for life, for your lifetime!

E.A.T.4life (Eat And Transform for life)
E.A.T.4life Eating Schedule

Before we begin, I want to issue a warning: This will seem so simple that you may be tempted to complicate it. Please do yourself a favor and *keep it simple*!

If you follow my program, you *will* get results. Below, I have listed *what to eat and when, serving sizes,* and a handy reference guide of *carbohydrates, vegetables, proteins, and fats.* As a bonus, I've added my official *Hit List* of foods to avoid.

Now remember, if you have been instructed by your nutritionist, naturopath, or doctor to avoid certain foods due to your specific health condition/concerns or body chemistry, *avoid those foods!* Not all bodies are alike and certain foods that may be healthful for the general population, may not be the best for you. If you have questions, speak with your health care provider or contact me at www.drshannonknows.com.

What to Eat and When

Breakfast: *2 Carbohydrates, 1 Protein (optional), 1 Vegetable (optional)* (Note: Yes, I know that vegetables are carbohydrates. However, I have listed them in their own category, except the ones that are highest in carbohydrates—see list below. I have done this because I believe that most people are severely lacking in daily vegetable intake, and in my opinion, everyone can benefit from eating more vegetables, especially the green ones! Unless you've been instructed by your doctor to avoid green vegetables due to a specific medical concern.)

Brunch: *1 Protein, 1 Carbohydrate, 1 Vegetable*

Lunch: *1 Protein, 1 Carbohydrate, 1 Vegetable*

Snack (before 3:00 p.m.): *1 Fruit or Vegetable*

Dinner: *1 Protein, 1 Vegetable (one that is higher in protein, if possible, but not necessary), 1 Carbohydrate/Protein (optional)*

Snack: *1 Protein that is higher in fat*

Fats can be added at any time throughout your day (see specific list below): *The daily serving equals one tablespoon*

Fresh water intake: *Half your body weight in ounces per day*

Eat approximately every 2-3 hours throughout the day

Serving Sizes

Each *carbohydrate, vegetable, and protein* should be *the size of your fist.* Each piece of *bread* should be *the size of your open hand. (Eat sparingly.)* For *fats,* the daily serving equals 1 tablespoon.

Carbohydrates, Vegetables, Proteins, and Fats

Carbohydrates

A. Fruit and Whole Grain Carbohydrates

Eat raw sprouted beans, rice, and grains whenever possible. Some of the benefits of sprouting include: more nutrients, less calories and carbohydrates, and increased protein availability.[10]

For those who are sensitive to gluten, I have put an * next to the gluten-free grains.

Rice

Brown rice

Wild rice

Whole grain pasta

Barley

Bulgar (cracked wheat)

Amaranth*

Rye

Spelt

Whole grain breads, cereals, and tortillas

Millet*

Buckwheat*

Grits

Steel Cut Oats
(Note: Oats are naturally gluten free, but may become contaminated with wheat during growing or processing.)

Quinoa*

Tomato

Apple

Strawberries

Blueberries

Blackberries

Raspberries

Cantaloupe

Honeydew melon

Watermelon

Banana

Apricot

Cherries

Fresh coconut

Plum

Yellow plum

Pluot

Kiwi

Grapefruit

Lime

Lemon

Peach

Pear

Orange

Tangerine

Clementine

Nectarine

Prune

Pineapple

B. Vegetables Highest in Carbohydrates

Corn

Potatoes

Squash

Yams

Sweet potatoes

Spaghetti squash

Carrots

C. Carbohydrates Highest in Proteins:
(referred to as Carbohydrate/Protein)

Chickpeas

Lentil beans

Lima beans

Garbanzo beans

Kidney beans

Black beans

Edamame

Pinto beans

White beans (Navy beans)

Vegetables

For your convenience, I've listed these vegetables according to their calcium content in descending order, with collard leaves containing the most. Fresh organic vegetable juice is great. (My favorite is fresh wheatgrass juice from my local Whole Foods store!) And of course, eat veggies in their raw, organic form as much as possible.

Collard (leaves)

Kale (leaves)

Collard (stems)

Parsley

Dandelion greens

Mustard greens

Kale (stems)

Beet greens

Broccoli

Fennel

Okra

Chives

Lettuce (loose-leaf)

Leek

Green onion

Artichoke

Red cabbage

Celery

Brussels sprouts

Garlic

Cucumber

Asparagus

Alfalfa sprouts

Arugula

Green beans

Spinach

Snap peas

Snow peas/peapods

Wheat grass

Zucchini

Beets

Cabbage lettuce

Cauliflower

Eggplant

Onions

Scallions

Parsnips

Jicama

Radish

Green/Red/Yellow peppers

Jalapeño pepper

Red/Green chiles

Soy sprouts

Turnip

Kohlrabi

Rutabaga

Basil

Cilantro

Proteins

A. Fish, Chicken, and More

When you eat fish, I recommend choosing wild instead of farm raised. Why? Studies show that farm-raised salmon contains high levels of polychlorinated biphenyl (PCB) and other contaminants that are linked to cancer and other health damage.[11] Overall, wild-caught fish are far superior, both nutritionally and environmentally, to farm-raised fish.[12] Due to potentially toxic mercury levels in the fish noted by asterisks in this list, it is recommended that you consume no more than three* or six** servings per month.[13]

Organic chicken breast

Organic turkey breast

Lean ground turkey

Dolphin-safe tuna (canned chunk light** or canned Albacore*)

Salmon

Cod (Alaskan)**

Ocean perch

Tilapia

Halibut (Pacific and Atlantic)**

Mahi Mahi**

Snapper**

Freshwater trout

Walleye

Whitefish

Lean, ground organic beef (Eat red meat very seldom)

Lean, top-sirloin steak (Eat red meat very seldom)

Organic, free-range chicken eggs (Eat only one yolk for every three egg whites)

B. Vegetables Highest in Protein

Alfalfa sprouts

Artichoke

Broccoli

Brussels sprouts

Collard (leaves)

Kale (leaves)

Green Leaf lettuce

Parsley

Spinach

Turnip greens

Beans: soybeans

C. Proteins High in Fat (Nuts and Seeds)

The serving size is a small handful. Nuts and seeds are best if they are soaked in water for a few hours before use. Doing so stimulates germination, increases the vitamin content, and may aid in digestion by neutralizing enzyme inhibitors and phytic acid.[14]

Almonds

Pine nuts

Flaxseeds

Macadamia nuts

Hazelnuts

Walnuts

Pumpkin seeds

Sesame seeds

Sunflower seeds

Fats

Sunflower oil

Sesame oil

Borage oil

Evening primrose oil

Marine lipids (molecularly distilled fish oils)

Extra-virgin, cold-pressed olive oil, grape seed oil, or flaxseed oil

Raw, organic almond butter

Avocado

Fresh coconut

Organic, extra-virgin coconut oil

Hit List (Foods to Avoid)

Pork

Shellfish

Artificial sweeteners

Hydrogenated oils

Fast food

Dairy products

Caffeine

Refined sugar

Table salt

White flour products

Additives, colorings, flavorings, preservatives (ie MSG or natural flavoring)

Palm oils

Vegetable oils (unless currently listed)

Nondairy creamers

Fruit juice (unless freshly juiced and in small quantity, only once a day, preferably in the morning)

Once a week, you get to exercise your "free-W.I.L.L. to eat" (free-**W**hatever **I** **L**ike/**L**ove to eat) by having a free-W.I.L.L. day. This means, whatever you would like to eat that isn't listed (except maybe on the Hit List), you are free to indulge in as you choose. Just remember, it's only one day a week!

If you would like to join our *health4life REVOLUTION!* and Be A REVOLUTION, please take your picture and measurements before (Week 1) and after (Week 12), and e-mail me your success stories. I can't wait to hear from you!

Go to www.drshannonknows.com to share your personal story of transformation!

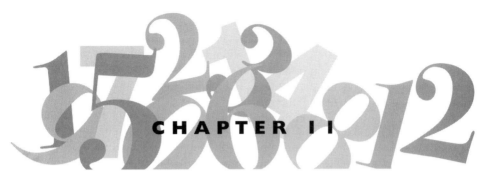

CHAPTER 11

Step #11: Train for Life

Did you know?

Any movement more than you are currently doing is considered exercise.

This chapter is all about *H.i.T.4life* (**H**igh **i**ntensity **T**raining for an incredible life). Don't let the word "intensity" scare you! I intentionally wrote it with a small letter "i" so it wouldn't be so intimidating.

"Intensity" means "the quality or state of being intense, especially strength, energy, or force,"[1] and "intense" is defined as "marked by great zeal, energy, or eagerness."[2] I believe we can all benefit from exercising more intensely and more intentionally. And you will be glad to know that I define exercise as an activity that is more than what you are doing right now. If you aren't used to walking much, walk. If you walk, walk more. If you walk more, jog or ride a bike. If you are used to sitting on a couch with a remote, get up to change the channel. Better yet, just get up off of that couch and move. Or watch TV while using your stationary bike and do resistance training during the commercials instead of going to the kitchen for a snack. If you usually take six steps, try taking twelve steps!

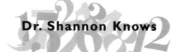

> *Where there is motion, there is life;*
>
> *and where there is life, there is motion.*

Change! It's really not as hard as you think. Start where you are and move forward. Transformation happens the moment you make a decision. Choose to exercise your right to exercise! We were designed to move or we wouldn't have joints and muscles. Where there is motion, there is life; and where there is life, there is motion. If you want to live, you must move. It's that simple.

In my practice, I have cared for a lot of hospice nurses. One day, I asked my nurse-patient how long it takes for a bedsore to set in. Her answer? Only four to five hours. (Can you believe that?) This is how important motion is to life and health in the body—every cell of it. You don't have to exercise every day for two hours to be healthy and fit. You can train as little as four hours a week and get fabulous results. Yes, it's true! Did you know that you can exercise and enjoy it? I dare you; it's your choice!

Several years ago, a woman named Marty attended my *H.i.T.* classes. She was very determined to get in shape and was always fun to have in class. During class one day, I noticed a look on her face of "Dear God, help me; I don't think I can do this anymore."

I very passionately and intensely reminded her that she could. "*Yes you can, Marty! Yes you can; you can do hard things!*" I yelled.

With a big, sweaty smile, she acknowledged me with an empowered look that said, "You know, you're right. Yes, I can. I can do hard things!" And she did! She finished the workout strong, and many more afterward.

That reminder became our class motto. *Yes you can; you can do hard things!* Think about it. If you've never trained before, let alone high-intensity trained before, don't be afraid. Today is your day to start. I will help you!

So often we think that exercise is working out at a gym for hours, or taking a fitness class, or running many miles. You can do those if you choose, but remember any movement more than you are currently doing is considered exercise. It sounds so simple, doesn't it? It is! It may not be easy, but it is simple. You can do hard things. H.A.R.D. can become E.A.S.Y. (Please see "Dr. Shannon's Defining Truths" after Step 12.)

Start somewhere and move.

One of my past clients was five hundred pounds and embodied this point. When he first began this program, he was barely able to walk up the steps to my studio. Within a few short weeks, he was not only moving up the steps quickly, but he wasn't using the handrails anymore, and he wasn't sweating and out of breath when he reached the top. When he exercised, he wasn't only walking, but he was running. After twelve short weeks, he had lost eighty-nine pounds and was happier than ever. None of this happened until he first decided to start somewhere and move.

We all have to start somewhere. The beauty of living a healthy, *wellthy* life is that we do it one step at a time.

H.i.T.4life
(High intensity Training for an incredible life)

Before you begin, walk over to your computer and go to www.drshannonknows.com and click "*health4life REVOLUTION!* High intensity Training Demos" to view detailed video demonstrations of each of the exercises. I want you to be very clear about what you are doing so you can move ahead with confidence.

Train on Monday, Wednesday, Friday, and Saturday or on Tuesday, Thursday, Saturday, and Sunday. Don't worry; you can schedule your training time as you can fit it in, but remember to allow a day between trainings (when possible) and no more than two consecutive training days in a row unless you are doing cardio only!

If your goal is significant weight loss, then add one or two additional sustained cardio training sessions each week. Do something fun and enjoyable: ride a bike, walk, jog, run, box, take a group fitness class, dance, or swim. (This could be your fifth or sixth training session of the week, if you choose.)

Equipment Needed:

Comfortable, supportive shoes: fitness or running depending on the cardio exercise of your choice

Jump rope (if you choose)

Bicycle: outdoor or stationary (if you choose)

Step (if you choose)

Treadmill (if you choose)

Heavy bag and boxing gloves (if you choose)

Pull-up bar (if you choose)

Weighted bar

Dumbbells

Exercise tube

Exercise band

Exercise ball

Exercise mat

Water bottle and towel

Your favorite high-energy music

<u>H</u>igh <u>i</u>ntensity <u>T</u>raining **Schedule:**

Please see below a concise schedule for your 60-minute workout. (If you do not have time to do 60 minutes, you can check out my 30-minute **H.i.T.** *Express* schedule on www.drshannonknows.com.) The lists that follow this schedule give you specific exercises to choose from for each segment of your training. Set up your cardio and strength training sessions before you begin so you are ready to go!

Warm-up:

Stationary biking, marching in place, walking, or light jump roping = 10 minutes

Alternate Cardio/Strength Stations*:

8 Cardio Stations for 3 minutes each (increase the intensity with each minute) = 24 minutes

Alternate with 8 Strength Stations for 1 minute each = 8 minutes (For example, do one cardio training exercise for 3 minutes followed by 1 minute of strength training. Then go to your next cardio station, followed by your next strength station, and so on.)

Total = 32 minutes

* Demonstrations of the following Cardio/Strength training can be viewed at www.drshannonknows.com.

Additional Leg Work/Additional Push-ups:

This can be performed after the warm-up before beginning specific Cardio/Strength Stations (women especially), or after the alternating Cardio/Strength Stations. You choose what works best for you. (My favorite is immediately after the warm-up.)

Total = 10 minutes

Stretching*:

At the end, stretch major muscle groups to cool down (hold each stretch for a minimum of 30 seconds each).

Finish with 8 deep breaths.

Total = 8 minutes

Total High intensity Training = 60 minutes

* Stretching demonstrations can be viewed at www.drshannonknows.com.

Cardio Stations:

Please choose 8 different exercises to create 8 stations, or choose 4 and repeat each for a total of 8 stations. Remember to use your arms as much as possible, especially when doing primarily lower body exercises like Marching in place, Knee lifts, High knees, Stepping side to side, Skipping, or Push kicks/Side kicks.

Running

Walking

Run/walk

Sprints

Biking

Boxing (cardio or heavy bag)

Jumping rope

Jumping jacks

Star jumps

Squat jumps

Split squat jumps

Burpees

Hops

Cross-countries

Crisscrosses

Shuffles

Lunges (side, back, front)

Knee lifts

High knees: running in place with knees up

Marching in place: pump arms, reach up/down, reach side/side, or side/down

Jogging in place

Stepping side to side

Skipping

Push kicks/ Side kicks

Stairs

Step-ups

Chatter feet (fast jogging in place, while keeping your feet very close to the floor)

Mountain climbers

Strength Stations:

Please alternate the 2 following Strength Sessions from below each time you train and choose 2 exercises per body part (unless otherwise instructed) from the following lists and alternate between each of the Cardio Stations. Remember, do 4 times per week on a rotating schedule of:

Strength Session One

Biceps

Triceps

Shoulders

Legs: Choose only 1 exercise

Abdominals: Choose only 1 exercise

Additional Leg Work using no weight: squats, lunges, walking lunges, leg lifts-front/side

Additional Push-ups (do 25, or more if you choose)

Strength Session Two

Chest

Back

Legs

Abdominals

Additional Leg Work using no weight: squats, lunges, walking lunges, leg lifts-front/side

Additional Push-ups (do 25, or more if you choose)

Biceps:

Curls with weighted bar

Curls with dumbbells: singles or doubles

Curls with exercise tube: singles or doubles

Hammer Curls with dumbbells: singles or doubles

Single-arm preacher curl on exercise ball

Triceps:

Triceps pushdown with exercise tube: singles or doubles over door/hinge (or pull-up bar)

Triceps press with exercise tube or dumbbells: overhead (single or double arms)

One-arm bent triceps extension with exercise tube or dumbbell

Dips (on the floor or step)

Triceps push-ups

Shoulders:
Shoulder press with dumbbells, weighted bar, or exercise tube
Lateral flyes with dumbbells or exercise tube
Bent-over flyes with dumbbells or exercise tube (posterior deltoids)

Legs: (exercise your legs with every training)
Squats with weighted bar, dumbbells, exercise tube, or no weight
Lunges with weighted bar, dumbbells, or no weight (front, side, or back)
Walking lunges with dumbbells or no weight
Standing lunges with exercise tube
Standing leg extensions with exercise tube under feet or band around ankles
Standing leg abductions with band around ankles (add a squat between alternate lifts)
Standing leg abductions with exercise tube (add a squat between alternate lifts)
Straight-leg dead lift with weighted bar or dumbbells
Standing calf raises on the floor or step
Side lying leg abductions or adductions with band around ankles
Prone leg curl with dumbbell between feet

Abdominals: (exercise your abdominals with every training)
Crunches: knees bent (can also be performed on exercise ball)
Crunches with oblique twist: knees bent (can also be performed on exercise ball)
Crunches: knees up
Crunches with oblique twist: knees up
Seated twists
Side-lying lifts
Planks
Side planks

Chest:
Push-up: on toes or knees (do with each of your 4 scheduled trainings)
Push-up with body on exercise ball
Chest press with weighted bar: on step, exercise ball, or floor
Chest press with dumbbell: on step, exercise ball, or floor
Dumbbell flyes on step, exercise ball, or floor
Standing exercise tube flyes: with or without tube connected to the door/hinge

Back:
Single arm pull-down with exercise tube
Pull-down with exercise tube over door/hinge (or pull-up bar)
Seated row with exercise tube
Upright row with dumbbells, weighted bar, or exercise tube
Bent-over row with weighted bar or dumbbells
Single-arm bent-over row with dumbbell
Pull-up: with or without assistance (with pull-up bar)
Pull-up with towel over door
Prone back extensions

Give yourself a big hug and a big hand. _You did it!_ You've completed eleven steps. Congratulations, you're almost there! How do you feel?

Did you know?
You create health and wellth while on the move!

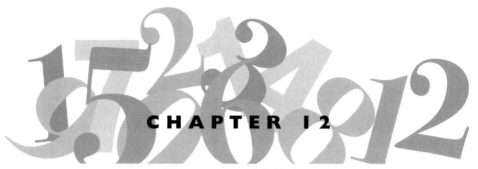

CHAPTER 12

Step #12:
Be a Revolution!

Did you know?
Your story has the power to change history!

Now that you've joined the movement, *BE A REVOLUTION!*

As you're walking out what you've learned in Steps #1 - #11, Step #12 is where you give back what you've received. By being the best *you* that you can be, and by sharing your story with others, you will be an answer to life's questions and a solution to life's problems for others—in short, you will *be a revolution*!

Revolution = a sudden, *radical*, or complete change.[1]

radical = *extreme*, a person who favors rapid and sweeping changes.[2]

extreme = very great or *intense*, going to great lengths or normal limits, utmost, maximum.[3]

intense = see the beginning of chapter 11. ☺

A revolution! = one who knows their *wellth* and prospers in health; one who dares to be the mission that begins with movement and continues with a message.

Your testimony holds infinite power. Tell everyone who will listen! As you share your story of health and *wellth*, people will be touched and lives will be transformed, including your own.

The message

I wrote this book because I believe I'm a messenger of hope, but I need your help. Will you be 1 in 1 million and do me a favor? If reading this book causes you to become more hopeful for a more prosperous tomorrow, please tell as many people as you can to read it and that they, too, can be healthy and *wellthy*. And please tell me; I would love to hear your story. You, too, have a message of hope to share.

The ultimate question is, what is the message you are living? May it be one of health for life. What kind of story is your life telling? May it be one of *wellth* and health for life.

Winston Churchill once said, "History will be kind to me for I intend to write it." Right now, you are writing not just your present, but your future. I believe we are here to touch people through telling our stories, and that is exactly what we will do. Together, we will make a difference! I personally invite you to join others in this movement as we inspire health and *wellth* while on the move! Just log on to www.drshannonknows.com, and BE A REVOLUTION!

As a part of something bigger than yourself, just watch the new movement in your life. Thank you for stepping into this revolution with me!

Revolutionary Stories

"I decided to join health4life because my weight inhibited every area of my life. Before health4life, I had no faith in myself and no hope for living out a long future. I now look forward to a vibrant life full of adventure. I've learned to accept peace in my life while embracing strength and vitality, and for the first time in my life—I am truly living."

—R.R., 2009 *health4life REVOLUTION!* Grand Champion
(Lost 25 pounds, 24 ¾ inches, and 7.3% body fat)

"Over the past several years, the youngest of my four children would call me 'her big fat daddy.' Then I would attempt to correct her, informing her that it was not nice to call another person fat, all the while knowing she was right. I was really a big fat daddy. This scenario, along with my lack of self-discipline during past diets, had me ready to get after it and make this health4life challenge a life-changing event. Many of the diets I had previously been on would concentrate mainly on losing weight without having to exercise. These would always go well for a while, then I would stop and gain more weight back than I had lost. The health4life challenge and its emphasis on exercising has brought me back in the gym and watching what I eat. Since I am exercising again, it seems that if I have a bad day with eating, I can make it up with an hour-long boot camp workout in the gym that gets me right back on track. Although it has been great to lose almost 40 pounds in 12 weeks, this program has done so much more for me. It has given me the ability to more easily tie my shoes, get outside and play with my kids after work, and be more energetic and interested in performing my daily work-related tasks. I have become more of a role model for my kids in eating the right foods and exercising on a routine basis."

—E.M.

"When I first started on this journey, I assumed this was going to be another failed attempt to lose weight. Why is it different now? I went to the first workout, and Dr. Shannon kicked my butt into gear. It opened my eyes to how out of shape I really was. Then the turning point…the first meeting, at which we were told to write out our goals. Mine was simple: 'LOSE WEIGHT.' Dr. Shannon said to really examine why we wanted to lose the weight, and it would happen. It was then I realized, I do not have an excuse to not lose weight, but every reason to push myself to do all I can to get healthy. I realized that this was my time, when talking about losing weight made me almost cry. I was not happy with who I was. I was unhappy and tried to hide it, so no one knew. I guess I did it well. So I went through the challenge, and celebrated every pound lost, because in the end it's not how much you lose, but the fact that you are doing something about it. I lost weight and inches; and while I am being honest, I have to tell you I also gained. I gained respect for myself, which I have not had in years. I gained confidence in myself that I let go of when I needed it most. I learned how to live a healthier lifestyle for myself and my daughter. I no longer hate the way I look. I still have some pounds to lose, but know I can look in the mirror and be happy with the Kristen I see. I am happy now, and want everyone to know it."

—K.V., 2011 *health4life REVOLUTION!* Grand Champion
(Lost 17 pounds and 24 ½ inches)

"My weight is something that I've always struggled with. Over the years I would lose weight, just to gain it all back in a few months. I had started losing weight before the challenge, but was halfheartedly trying. My trainer mentioned the health4life challenge because I needed some motivation to lose weight. Joining the challenge was hard for me. I did not want anyone else knowing my weight. Any time I have had to mention my weight, I break down crying because I can't believe I have gained so much. While writing my goals and reasons for wanting to lose weight, I decided that this was my new beginning: I'm tired of my weight keeping me from doing things I want in life or want to try; if I start now, then I will be healthy enough to do things later. My first step was to work out more. A lady had been inviting me to a Zumba dance class, but I thought, 'I just can't do it, I'm too overweight.' I actually enjoy working out. The hardest thing for me has been changing my eating habits. It's so easy to go back to old eating habits, especially when I'm stressed. I have been able to go to my favorite restaurant and choose something healthy. Joining health4life is just the beginning of my weight-loss journey. It's not just a 12-week challenge, but a lifestyle change."

—S.U. (Lost 32 pounds and 21 ½ inches)

Before health4life challenge

"I am always crabby. When I look at myself, I feel disgusted. My thighs rub together. My clothes are tight. I am not happy at all! I would like to feel healthy and happy…I am ready to make a change."

After health4life challenge

"I look in the mirror and see a beautiful woman. I can tell myself, 'I love you!' This isn't conceit; it's hard to explain. Back in January (12 weeks ago), I was so disgusted with myself. Today, I don't understand why I felt that way. How could anyone feel like that? How sad! I lost 6.1% body fat and 15 pounds. That's a lot of fat! Twelve weeks—amazing!! My only goal is to stay happy and healthy. By staying on this path, the fat will burn away! Thank you, Dr. Shannon."

—L.N.

"When I started, I weighed 178 pounds…my total weight loss is 20 pounds. Although I am not a fitness guru now, I am an expert in one thing and this is being ME. When I started this program, I was in GREAT DENIAL. I thought I could teach myself how to eat right and exercise and yet every year…no change, no progress. Now I know that the competition never mattered, the winning wasn't important; it was the wisdom I gained that has made me victorious! A big thanks to Dr. Shannon…she was amazingly supportive and positive every day. It can only get better from here!"

—R.B.

"I actually lost twenty pounds and lowered my body fat…I feel I can truly achieve any and all new goals that I set for myself!"

—D.H.

"health4life helped me start treating my body more like a temple instead of a barn."

—M.N., 2002 *health4life REVOLUTION!* Grand Champion

"When I first began this journey, something immediately changed. Blinders were taken off. Previously, I had looked at myself compared to others my size and thought, 'That's not me. I'm not like them.' Immediately after starting, I realized that I did need to change my body and lifestyle. Getting proper perspective of my physical appearance was a huge motivator. Once I made the decision that this was my time to change, unhealthy foods and drinks that were previously part of my normal diet became easy for me to resist. I haven't had one soda since I started this journey. I have realized that I really don't need the things that were once a problem. Another thing that I realized was that I needed to increase my self-talk. Having a team to encourage you is important, but when no one is around, you need to be able to encourage yourself. When I was running mile after mile or lifting weights, I had to say to myself, 'You can do this or you got this, this is easy, or you've already run 2 miles at this pace, another mile is no problem.' As a result of this challenge, I have become a new person. My outside body has changed dramatically, but it is the inner change that is the most significant."

—K.W., 2010 *health4life REVOLUTION!* Grand Champion
(Lost 40 pounds and 24 ¾ inches)

"My goal as I started the health4life challenge was to lose some weight. But God had bigger plans! Through chiropractic care, I realized that I can have a healthy body, long term. The greatest achievement over the last 12 weeks is being able to prepare myself for my calling."

—J.H., 2007 *health4life REVOLUTION!* Grand Champion
(Lost 21 pounds and 28 ¼ inches in just 12 weeks!)

"Through the health4life contest, I have lost nearly 20 pounds of fat, almost 9% of fat, and gained 7 pounds of muscle in 12 weeks! My soul has lifted and I am FREE—free of nasty habits that were killing me physically and spiritually—free to do the things I've dreamed of doing."

—M.O., 2003 *health4life REVOLUTION!* Grand Champion
(Lost 20 pounds and 9% of body fat)

"I have lost almost 40 pounds and over 22 inches in 12 weeks! I am so fired up and excited about the…probability that I will reach my 100-pound weight loss goal by the end of the summer. I recommitted myself to begin respecting and honoring that temple that God has entrusted me with. This program has been life changing for myself and my wife…"

—N.D., 2008 *health4life REVOLUTION!* Grand Champion
(Lost 39 pounds and 22.5 inches)

"I set out to try and improve my lifestyle so that it would include exercise and a healthier diet. I really feel that I have achieved that and more in 12 weeks. My goal is to be around, not just for my children, but also for my grandchildren, which is something my father did not do. The health4life program was never about a number on a scale for me. It is not a results-measured success that I was after. I have always been after the effort. I really feel like I put in a strong, consistent effort…and as a result of that effort, over the course of 12 weeks, I lost 50 pounds. I don't intend to stop here. I feel better than I have in a very long time."

—M.G.

"Before health4life: At 41, I feel like a tired, old, fat man with pain in my feet and an ache in my heart, which has led to alcoholism and depression. I am sickened and disgusted by my current physical, emotional, and financial conditions and wish to rip that dark, heavy cloak off…. It is time for my comeback.

"After health4life: I no longer eat and drink myself into a stupor every night. I have positive goals now … I have new friends, a better posture, a positive attitude, and my zest for life back. I am proud of what I have been able to accomplish the past 12 weeks. It's the longest I have ever stuck with such a commitment. I am going to continue down this path. After all, it's 'health4…LIFE, right?'"

—D.N.

"I am what I am and what I am is WONDERFUL! Thanks!"

—J.Z.

"When I started health4life 12 weeks ago, I weighed two pounds more than I did when I was nine months pregnant. My clothes were too tight. I was basically uncomfortable in my own skin. I had my daughter take my first week's pictures. When I saw myself, I felt even worse! I thought about giving up right then. I am so glad I didn't! I thought I would never show anyone the pictures from the first week, but when I saw the pictures from the twelfth week, I felt more proud of what I had done with myself than ashamed of what I used to be. I am so glad I did health4life. I learned a lot…I am thrilled with the results and I'm excited about my new way of life."

—P.M.

"All I can think of is how happy I am of what I accomplished in 12 weeks. I'm doing things that I've never dreamed of. For example, I recently bought some running shoes thinking I would try a jog around the block, and now I'm up to 3 miles! It's fun! I lost more weight than I thought, and gained muscle! My arms are not noodles anymore! My aches are gone and my pants are baggy in the legs and butt. My husband noticed and that is a great feeling. At the beginning I was so frustrated, and thought I'd never make it. How close I was to quitting…it's out of the question! This experience has helped me in other areas too. I have energy now to face things that I procrastinated doing…dealing with everyday stress is not so bad now. I don't know where this journey is leading me, but I'm enjoying the trip!"

—M.K.

"With the health4life competition ending, I find myself at the beginning of a wonderful lifelong journey. I am on the right path of monitoring my food intake, participating in a consistent exercise routine, and engaging in positive self-talk. Through this experience I have lost body fat, and equally important, I have lost ALL my previous excuses for not following through with my resolutions to become healthy and fit. I have learned what it means to be committed to myself and how that commitment translates into success."

—L.W. (Lost 16 pounds and 24 inches in 12 weeks)

"During the 12-week challenge, I have learned how to eat sensibly and what foods to avoid. I plan ahead when things get busy. As a woman, I now see the benefits of strength training and it is something I do regularly. Each week I am losing weight and getting stronger, and I am into pants I haven't worn in two years. My husband has noticed the change and calls me 'slim.' I have developed a permanent lifestyle of eating healthy and regular exercise."

—T.H. (Lost 12 pounds and 21 ½ inches in 12 weeks)

"The past 12 weeks have been amazing. My journey began two years ago when I stepped on a scale and realized that I weighed over 300 pounds! Right then, I decided that I needed to take control of my life and that is exactly what I did! Over the past two years, my lifestyle has been completely transformed. I have to admit, it has been the hardest thing I have ever done, yet the most rewarding. My eating habits have improved greatly and I actually enjoy and look forward to exercising! In the past two years, I have lost a grand total of 111 pounds! At my biggest, I wore a size 26 in clothing and now I am a size 12! Sometimes I can't even believe it! I had to realize that no one could do it for me but ME! I felt like the weight had kept me from living the life that God wants me to live! I was extremely unhealthy, and very unhappy. I now look forward to the rest of my life and embrace the new 'ME'!"

—S.D.

"I signed up for the health4life Challenge for a different reason. I had been going through a divorce and the sadness had become overwhelming. I was consumed by the thoughts of loss all day, and my self-esteem was almost nothing. I had met Dr. Shannon a few times for 30 minutes of inspiration on my lunch breaks. The power of her message during those lunch talks began to give me hope that there would be something good in my life again, but I was the one responsible for finding it. When Dr. Shannon told me about the health4life Challenge, I signed up in hopes of learning more from her about overcoming the challenge I was facing. Attending the workshops was where I expected to gain the most from the program. I knew Dr. Shannon could point the way to a better life. And she did. I just never expected the depth of change that I experienced. It is not what I lost that really matters. It is what I have gained. Spiritually and emotionally, I am a hopeful, confident, and determined woman. I have learned that through faith I can accomplish whatever goals I set for myself. And my goal is to be my best. I feel good. And I know that eating the right foods and adding exercise to my day plays a huge part in that. My body has let me know that it likes to move and it likes to be pushed to its limit. Exercise will forever be a part of my life. My greatest changes have occurred inside. To believe that you have a 'best' is empowering. Thanks, Dr. Shannon."

—B.W.

"Dr. Shannon emphasized to me the importance of commitment, consistency, and allowing the weight to come off naturally without a quick fix. As I began to commit to the program, I have noticed a slow, gradual change over a period of time. This program introduced me to High intensity Training, the proper way to maintain and lose weight; and, praise the Lord, I don't have to starve myself to be thin!"

—F.H.

"I was experiencing depression and had become somewhat reclusive. No matter how hard I tried to get "things" under control, I got nowhere. My husband tried to help me, but I would shrug him off. Remember the story of the man who was sitting on his roof during a flood praying to God for help? Every time help would come, he pushed it away saying God would help him…that was me 12 weeks ago. That is why I know in my heart that the health4life program was a lifesaver from God. We were asked to write our goals for the next 12 weeks. So I did: lose 10 pounds, eat regularly, and exercise. What happened was my WHOLE body shrank! I've dropped 2 pant sizes! I began eating according to the food list. My workouts involve High intensity Training and yoga 2 days. I've experienced incredible results. Not only has my body changed inside and out, I no longer experience depression or feeling reclusive. The success I feel in my heart goes far beyond what I can express in words. Thank you, God. And thank you, Dr. Shannon."

—D.C.

"This challenge for fitness has been an eye-opener. My nutrition has been life changing, not a diet. I have been drinking 6-8 bottles of water DAILY and I can see the difference. My life has been enriched the most by the challenge of my Accountability Partner. We talk daily and discuss what we ate. So many days ice cream was calling my name, but I refused because I did not want to confess to my Accountability Partner. We plan to continue and I thank you for the program."

—A.M.

"Weight has been an ongoing wrestling match since age 14. I, like many, have the ability to push myself towards fitness goals and lose weight, but I also, like the majority, have the ability to put back on what I have taken off. It is my choice. I choose whether I will be fat or fit! I have decided to, in the words of Dr. Shannon, 'Chase after optimum health, before sickness and disease chase after me.' I have decided that I have only one life to live on this earth and I am on a personal journey to discover what my 'personal best' looks like and live to that standard. Thank you, Dr. Shannon! I appreciate you being honest with me, speaking words of TRUTH that have pushed me to act out on my desire for better! Dr. Shannon, I appreciate you meeting me by the 'side of the road,' and looking past my exterior and seeing the best in me. I felt like you literally looked past my faults and saw what I needed."

—F.H. (Lost 17 pounds and 17 ¾ inches in 12 weeks)

"This challenge has drastically transformed me in such a way that every area of my life has been impacted. I praise God for the opportunity to be a part of this amazing program. Before health4life I was ill, unhappy with my image, and 40 pounds overweight. I was sick for the past 5 years with irregular menstrual cycles, headaches, and emotional mood swings. Last March, I was diagnosed with polycystic ovarian syndrome. My doctor said it was due to being overweight. So this is why I joined the competition; in hopes of bringing my body to health so that my husband and I can have a baby. My PCOS has completely gone away. I am only 10 pounds from reaching my goal. I am excited because I know I am capable of reaching my goals. What I learned from the workshops helped me to be a better friend, wife, and most importantly, a better Christian. It is my responsibility to take care of my temple to honor God. My temple is now FIT. FIT to honor God, FIT to help others, and FIT to be a mom! Thank you, Doc."

—M.T.

"Because of this program my spirit, soul, and body are in the process of being happy, healthy, and holy! Thanks, Dr. Shannon."

—A.A.

"After telling a friend that I was overweight, she looked at me and said, 'Well, you hide it really well!' At first I took it as a compliment, but then that's the moment I realized, 'I don't want to hide anymore.' I was tired of buying larger-sized clothes to hide areas of excess fat overflowing my jeans. I was sick of getting bigger and my clothes getting tighter. I was tired of being tired all the time and having no energy. This was the time to actually do something about it. Thus, the journey of health4life began. I am not sure what it was, but something inside of me just kicked into gear. I already felt like a brand-new person just getting started. As I began to eat right and work out more often, I noticed that I stayed full all day and had so much energy. I couldn't believe it! It feels so great to actually have old clothes fit better, while other clothes are so loose that they are about to fall off me. Even T-shirts that used to be tight on me are big and baggy. While I am physically dropping in size, I am emotionally increasing in self-esteem and confidence. I know that I am healthy. And I know that I have created a lifestyle, not just a diet or program that I can continue to follow and stay healthy. I am healthy. I am energized. Thank you for giving me this opportunity to challenge myself and push through. It has been hard work and it has paid off! Thank you for believing in me."

— A.H. (Lost 17 pounds and 19 inches in 12 weeks)

"At the age of 15, I began to struggle with my body image; although I had never been overweight, I felt as if I was much bigger than many of my friends. At some point, I felt as if dieting and exercise were just not enough and I began to binge and purge. I joined health4life because I thought I needed a quick fix to my fast, 30-pound gain. I never thought in a million years this program would change my life. Now only 12 weeks into this life-long program, I feel as if I can conquer anything. I have full control over my eating and that is the best feeling in the world, a feeling I had never experienced. I am very blessed that I had the opportunity to join health4life. I am my B.E.S.T. self! Thank you, Dr. Shannon."

— A.F. (Lost 21 ½ pounds and 19 ¼ inches)

"I began this journey with health4life weighing over 500 pounds. My family doctor had told me 3 months prior that he didn't expect me to live 10 years without dramatic weight loss and lifestyle changes. I was also being treated for ulcer-like wounds on my shins that weren't healing. The wound specialist informed me I was a good candidate for amputation. I was placed in the prescreening stages for gastric bypass surgery. I really didn't want to have surgery, but couldn't think of alternatives. Dieting had never given me long-term results; in fact, I believe dieting got me in the situation I was in. Enter heatlth4life and Dr. Shannon...I was a pretty serious project since my mobility and capacity to exercise were severely limited. Initially, we couldn't even find a scale capable of weighing me. The nutrition program started before the exercise, as I had to be cleared by my family doctor. I did my first workout. It wasn't much, and it hurt, but I had started. We arbitrarily guessed my starting weight at 500 pounds, although it could have been as much as 530-550 pounds. I am now at 419 pounds and have been losing consistently 5 ½ to 7 pounds per week. I know this is working because I am NOT dieting. I don't count calories or measure portions. I DO eat sensibly, but I don't feel like I am depriving myself of anything. There's no 'I can't eat that until I am done with this diet' mind-set. As far as the exercise…every day I feel stronger and more flexible. I can walk and stand for extended periods of time without fatigue. My feet don't hurt like they did. My blood pressure has dropped markedly. My clothes are falling off. People tell me I 'look healthier.' I don't have to ask people to do things for me all the time. I'm sleeping better. The wounds on my shins are almost gone! My resting pulse rate is 60 bpm, and the workouts—I can actually run! I haven't been able to run in YEARS! The workouts are still WORK, and always will be, but the benefits in everything else I do in my life are worth it. My deepest and heartfelt thanks to Dr. Shannon and all the staff at cornerstone4health CHIROPRACTIC. And finally, I'd like to thank God for showing me He's not ready for me yet…"

—T.B. (Lost 81+ pounds in just 12 short weeks)

"I thank God that my wife told me about health4life because it has changed my life! When I signed up for this challenge, I had two goals: to get a ripped body and prove to myself that I could be consistent at something besides procrastinating. More than anything, I wanted to look good in my T-shirts this summer. My muscles have grown and I have more energy than I've had since high school. I also proved to myself that I could be consistent with a workout regimen. This was a huge accomplishment for me because I never worked out on my own for more than two weeks. The workshops were so inspirational. They kept me focused on my goals and helped me change the way that I think. My mind-set went from 'I can't' to 'I can and I will.' Even the weeks that I didn't feel like working out or didn't stick to my schedule, I never condemned myself or gave up. I really believe that God used this program to strengthen my mind. Being healthy is becoming a lifestyle and my determination and passion for life are stronger than ever!"

—W.C.

"I am 38 years old and have struggled with my weight for most of my life. It seems I have been on every diet imaginable, but could never succeed at any one of them for very long. Once embarking on my health4life journey, there seemed to be many obstacles trying to get in the way, so I tried to attend as many workshops as possible. They were so inspirational, and had so many nuggets of information that once really absorbed, were virtually life changing. The one that stood out most to my husband and me was the one on making the decision to be healthy and to exercise. Dr. Shannon shared that when you make a decision, the translation of 'decision' is to actually cut off any other options of failure. Wow! That was so eye-opening for me. How many times had I thought I had decided to do some-thing, but still left the back door open for many distractions that could pull me away from what I was trying to do in my life? Too many to count, that is for sure. There are days when I feel like I am at the starting line again, but I always try to remember: Being Excellent Starting Today, and I can be my B.E.S.T. I need to find contentment deep inside and know who I am in Christ, and that God did not create junk! I CAN like what I see in the mirror, instead of letting that mirror reflect how the enemy wants me to see myself. I am daily learning to awaken the warrior within! I have to learn that it does not matter who sees me, as I have always been ashamed to get out and exercise; always being the 'fat girl' but I am not only transforming my mind, but my body also. I can't transform my body unless I exercise. I am also daily shedding the victim mentality, and am arising the warrior! I have found that by digging deep inside to my inner being, as scary as it's been, I am starting to like what's inside. Here I am at the end of this 12-week journey, but the journey is still ongoing every day of my life, and with all the valuable information from the workshops instilled in my mind, I feel strong inside and out, mentally, physically, and spiritually. I know that this process is a journey and I am learning to take each day for what it is—a gift from God—and live it to the fullest!"

—K.C.

"Through a major transition in my life (divorce/loss) I chose food to comfort me, and to become physically and emotionally unhealthy. I thought, 'I want to do something different. I'm tired of being unhealthy and being a bad example for my children.' (They were choosing food to comfort themselves, as well.) Through the process of this challenge, I have learned that it is daily choices that make a difference. I was my own worst enemy, beating myself up over wrong choices. My daily life is different now. My children make better food choices because of the changes I have made. I have made it through the 'challenge' despite obstacles such as a car accident and losing my job. I am proud of myself! I don't feel like this challenge is over; I actually feel like I've just begun. Fat/weight loss is only a small part of the transformation that has occurred in my life. It feels so good to be emotionally and physically healthy. Thanks, health4life!" ☺

—K.S. (Lost 30 pounds and 14 ½ inches)

"When building a home, one begins with a foundation for the home to stand upon. In this transformation I learned that I had an extremely weak, shoddy, poor foundation, which is why I would lose and regain weight constantly. Our foundation is to be love, but for me I could love others, but not Andrea. One night on my way to Dr. Shannon's workshop, I heard a still, small voice: 'Andrea, you don't love yourself.' That hit me like a ton of bricks. I pulled over and cried. I would help others, buy for others, but I was not good enough to invest in myself. I was not worth it. This program taught me that I am worth it. In the last 90 days, my guilt over my sister's death was removed. For 32 years I have not lived life to the fullest because of this weight. Dr. Shannon gave me the keys to get out of the prison cell;

she opened the door. She did what she could, but I am the only one who could make that decision to step out of cell number '289.' I will be 50 years old on September 7. Actress Valerie Bertinelli is on the cover of *Good Housekeeping*, looking beautiful and healthy. The cover states, 'This is what 50 looks like.' Fifty means jubilee, which means freedom! Yes, 50 will look good on me because of the inner transformation. Outer transformation without inner is only temporary. But God showed me my problem, which was a lack of love for Andrea, and things began to change. Has it been easy to learn to love myself? No, but it is possible. I owe it to God and my fellow man to be the best I can be. As long as I keep success in my vocabulary, the weight will continue to melt as I have changed my eating habits. Instead of craving sweets, I crave black olives and tilapia! Thank you, Dr. Shannon, for keeping me focused and accountable."

—A.A. (Lost 20 pounds and 8 inches)

"As I look back over the past three months, I have seen many changes within myself. I had a difficult time in the beginning, grasping all the mental and physical aspects of the challenge. However, it did not take long until I could feel myself welcoming the changes in my body. One of the first challenges was to give up drinking diet soda. That was very hard for me. I began to drink only water and could tell a big difference very quickly. Throughout the health4life workshops, I gained a new knowledge of how important good nutrition is for my body. I now know how necessary it is to take the time to plan ahead, and be aware of all the ingredients in the food that we eat. I have increased my endurance, become stronger mentally and physically, and have developed a new appreciation of myself as a whole person. Since I started this journey, I have rediscovered my love of running. Through all this, I have made many new friends and have realized that accountability equals success. All my life I have been self-conscious about my body. This process has helped me tremendously, and I now feel much more self-assured and confident. By far, the most dramatic changes for me during this time have been mental more than physical. My family and friends have all noticed a big difference in my outlook on life and my self-esteem. I now have the courage to feel good about myself. Having seen such positive changes in my life, I would certainly, with no hesitation, recommend others begin looking for those changes in themselves. By participating in health4life, other people can begin the process of achieving their personal goals in body, mind, and spirit."

—B.W. (Lost 7 pounds and 12 inches)

"When I began this journey, I 'wanted' to lose weight. My entire adult life I have 'wanted' to lose weight. Today, I 'desire' to continue my weight-loss journey. Over the past several weeks, my mind-set has changed to BELIEVE I can achieve my goals. Rather than viewing today as the end of the challenge, I simply see it as a checkpoint on my map. Throughout the challenge, I have achieved the following: I have changed the shape of my body; I no longer need the antidepressant I've been taking for over three years; I am no longer addicted to caffeine; I no longer take naps in the afternoons because I'm too tired to make it through the day; I no longer plan my days around food; I have embraced exercise; I have claimed control of my life; I have thrown away my 'fat' clothes; I refuse to be a part of the 95% of people who lose weight only to gain it back; and, I have adopted a new lifestyle. As a result, my bond with my husband is stronger. I like him more because I like ME more. My relationship with my children is more fun. I can enjoy activities with them instead of being too tired to participate. My relationship with myself has changed. I stop to look in mirrors now. I shop for fitted clothes. Most importantly, my relationship with God has changed. I no longer feel ashamed of what I've done to His temple, but feel eager to make better choices every day."

—S.K. (Lost 23 pounds and 13 ¼ inches)

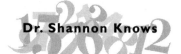

"I truly have been transformed inside and out from this program. Thank you for health4life!"

—R.N.

"I've lived in fear my whole life. It's been generational. I've watched my parents do it and their parents. I didn't even know that I had a choice. I am so excited about the possibilities that are available to me! Thank you so much for giving me such hope. I had no idea!"

—One of my patients, after reading the first three steps of the manuscript of this book

What is the key to change?

The key to transformation is renewing your mind. You (and I) can always go back to Step #1 and any of them in between when we need to. The Bible says that we are "transformed by the renewing of [our] mind."[4] What does "renew" mean? "To make or become new, fresh, or strong again, *revive*, to make or do again: *repeat*, to begin again: *resume*."[5] Going back and doing these steps over and over again for a lifetime would constitute a "renewing of our minds," and therefore, bring us a life of transformation, health, and *wellth*.

Remember, *you* are the revolution!

I cannot wait to hear your story! Go to www.drshannonknows.com to share it. I look forward to hearing from you!

Now you *KNOW*,

Dr. Shannon and all those who *know* their *wellth*

DR. SHANNON'S DEFINING TRUTHS

A.D.I.O. = **A**bove **D**own **I**nside **O**ut

A Revolution = One who knows their *wellth* and prospers in health; one who dares to be the mission that begins with movement and continues with a message.

Be 1 of 11 = Be a Partner

Be a Celebrity = Be *greatful* (No, not a typo.)

Be Answerable = Be responsible

Be a Revolution! = Be healthy, Be *wellthy*, Be the solution, Be "his (or her) story"; inspiring health and *wellth* while on the move!

B.E.S.T. = **B**e **E**xcellent **S**tarting **T**oday

Be Question-able = Ask questions

Be Your B.E.S.T. from A.D.I.O. = Be the way God designed you to be, healthy, *wellthy*

E.A.S.Y. = an **E**xcellent **A**nd **S**uccessful **Y**ou

E.A.T.*4life* = **E**at **A**nd **T**ransform for life

Eat Responsibly…For Life = Eat to live, *not* live to eat

Exercise = an activity that is more than what you are doing right now, a celebration of the ability to move

Expose Yourself = Face your fears

Faith = what I base my life on

Fear = Anything standing in the way of my health and *wellth*

Free-W.I.L.L. to eat = (free-**W**hatever **I** **L**ike/**L**ove to eat)

Greatful = Gratitude that causes a state of being filled with greatness

H.A.R.D. (How hard can become E.A.S.Y.) = **H**ave a Health Plan, **A**bundance Thinking, be **R**adical, make a **D**ecision…and become an **E**xcellent **A**nd **S**uccessful **Y**ou

H.I.T. = **H**ope, **I**nspiration, **T**iming

H.i.T.4life = **H**igh **i**ntensity **T**raining for an incredible life, an exercise program that will transform your body and your life

Health = Full expression of life

health4life REVOLUTION! (aka health4life) = a health and fitness opportunity that will challenge the participants to not only join the revolution, but be the revolution; proven, effective eating and exercise program that empowers individuals to be their best (see Step #12 for detailed stories of defining health4life)

Healthy = Experiencing and enjoying the *full* expression of life (and *wellth*) that's on the inside of you: *best*

K.N.O.W. = **K**now **N**ow **O**r **W**ant

Know Yourself = Dare to Desire

L.T.O. = **L**ess **T**han **O**ptimal, symptomatic, but overcoming (aka: I am healing); something to say the next time you feel not so well

Locate Yourself = Admittance

Messenger of Hope = Dr. Shannon and *you* as well, once you complete Step #12

Recovery = Your rightful healing

"the nspirer" = an inspiring message of hope for minds that want to grow and those who want to know (YouTube- thenspirer)

Train for Life = Play to win instead of playing *not* to lose

True health and wealth = *wellth*

Valuably Free = Freedom

Well…come = an invitation to experience the truth, speak the truth, know the truth, and live the truth…and your *well* will come.

Wellth = True health and wealth; the physical (body, mind, and spirit) embodiment of the fiscal definition of wealth. Or quite simply, it's the wealth inside of you; wealth in your body. Your *wellth* is the source of your health!

(FYI: Once you become truly *wellthy*, your economic value will increase as well. ("Wealth" = "all objects or resources that have an economic value" (*Merriam-Webster's* is so smart!)

Wellthy = The wealth on the inside of you being fully expressed in your body, mind, spirit, and life: *best*

Wonder = Why I began to write this book

Hmm, I *wonder* what my next book will be about? I just wonder! ☺

NOTES

Preface

1. *Franklin Merriam-Webster's Dictionary & Thesaurus*, 2004, s.v. "Wonder."
2. "America's Health Checkup," *TIME*, November 20, 2008.
3. Ibid.
4. *Twelve Steps and Twelve Traditions*, (New York: Alcoholics Anonymous and World Services, Inc., 2007).
5. *Franklin Merriam-Webster's Dictionary & Thesaurus*, 2004, s.v. "Recovery."
6. Ibid., s.v. "Wealth."
7. Ibid.
8. Ibid., s.v. "Best."
9. Ibid., s.v. "Well."

Before You Begin

1. Matthew 7:13-14 New International Version.
2. "America's Health Checkup," *TIME*, November 20, 2008.
3. http://drugwarfacts.org/cms/?q=node/30.
4. http://www.justice.gov/dea/concern/prescription_drug_fact_sheet.html.

5. http://www.cdc.gov/HomeandRecreationalSafety/Poisoning/brief.html.

6. www.foxnews.com/story/0,2933,362681,00.html.

7. Ibid.

8. http://products.sanofi-aventis.us/ambien/ambien.pdf, 5-6.

9. http://www.cbsnews.com/stories/2002/11/14/sunday/main529388.shtml.

10. Ibid.

11. http://nutritionbusinessjournal.com/healthy-foods/news/08-05-cbs-news-com-reports-caffeine-intoxication-rise/.

12. Based on data drawn from the 2007 World Population Data Sheet, hoovers.com and Euromonitor "The World Market for Consumer Foodservice, 2004." http://www.suite101.com/content/top-fast-food-countries-a29881.

13. http://articles.mercola.com/sites/articles/archive/2010/04/20/sugar-dangers.aspx.

14. http://digestive.niddk.nih.gov/ddiseases/pubs/constipation/.

15. http://www.intermartialarts.com/article/sumo-wrestler-diet.

16. Luke 6:37 New International Version.

17. *Franklin Merriam-Webster's Dictionary & Thesaurus,* 2004, s.v. "Settle," Definition #14.

Chapter 1, Step 1: Expose Yourself

1. Philippians 2:9.

2. Hebrews 11:1 New King James Version.

3. John 8:32 New International Version.

4. *Franklin Merriam-Webster's Dictionary & Thesaurus,* 2004, s.v. "Hope."

5. Hebrews 11:1 New International Version.

6. *Franklin Merriam-Webster's Dictionary & Thesaurus,* 2004, s.v. "Sure."

7. Ibid., s.v. "Certain."

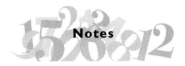

8. Proverbs 13:17 New Living Translation.

9. *Franklin Merriam-Webster's Dictionary & Thesaurus*, 2004, s.v. "HOPE."

Chapter 2, Step 2: Locate Yourself

1. Genesis 3:1 New International Version.

2. Genesis 2:16-17 New International Version.

3. Genesis 3:4 New International Version.

4. Genesis 3:5 New International Version.

5. Genesis 3:6 New International Version.

6. Genesis 3:9 New International Version.

Chapter 3, Step 3: Know Yourself

1. Psalm 37:4 New International Version.

2. *Franklin Merriam-Webster's Dictionary & Thesaurus*, 2004, s.v. "Want."

3. Ibid., s.v. "Desire."

4. Ibid., s.v. "Desiderare."

5. Jeremiah 1:5 New International Version.

6. 1 John 4:18 New International Version.

Chapter 4, Step 4: Be Answerable

1. *Franklin Merriam-Webster's Dictionary & Thesaurus*, 2004, s.v. "Responsibility."

2. Ibid., s.v. "Serve."

3. Proverbs 13:17 New Living Translation.

4. *Franklin Merriam-Webster's Dictionary & Thesaurus*, 2004, s.v. "In the know."

5. Ibid., s.v. "Confidential."

6. Ibid., s.v. "Confidence."

7. Proverbs 13:17 New Living Translation.

Chapter 5, Step 5: Be a Celebrity

1. *Franklin Merriam-Webster's Dictionary & Thesaurus,* 2004, s.v. "Celebrity."

2. Ibid., s.v. "Capriccio."

Chapter 7, Step 7: Be Question-able

1. Romans 10:9 New Living Translation.

2. Matthew 12:34 New King James Version.

3. Romans 10:17 New King James Version.

4. *Franklin Merriam-Webster's Dictionary & Thesaurus,* 2004, s.v. "Decide."

5. Mark 10:27 New King James Version.

Chapter 8, Step 8: B.E.S.T. from A.D.I.O.

1. Genesis 1:31 New International Version.

2. "America's Health Checkup," *TIME,* November 2010.

3. http://www.whale.to/a/null9.html#ABSTRACT.

4. http://www.whale.to/a/null9.html#Table_3:_Estimated_10-Year_Death_Rates_from_Medical_Intervention.

5. Ibid.

6. *Franklin Merriam-Webster's Dictionary & Thesaurus,* 2004, s.v. "Best."

7. Ibid., s.v. "Well."

Chapter 9, Step 9: Be 1 of 11

1. *Franklin Merriam-Webster's Dictionary & Thesaurus,* 2004, s.v. "Answerable."

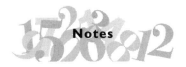

Chapter 10, Step 10: Eat Responsibly for Life!

1. http://www.marketsandmarkets.com/Market-Reports/global-weight-loss-and-gain-market-research-28.html.

2. http://www.veghealthguide.com/nuts-seeds/.

3. http://ezinearticles.com/?Benefits-of-Sprouted-Foods&id=114242.

4. en.wikipedia.org, s.v. "Pesticide residue."

5. http://www.thedailygreen.com/healthy-eating/eat-safe/Dirty-Dozen-Foods.

6. http://www.foodnews.org/sneak/EWG-shoppers-guide.pdf.

7. Ibid.

8. Ibid.

9. http://articles.cnn.com/2010-06. 01/health/dirty.dozen.produce.pesticide_1_pesticide-residue-pesticide-tests-fruits-and-vegetables?_s= PM:HEALTH.

10. http://ezinearticles.com/?Benefits-of-Sprouted-Foods&id=114242.

11. http://www.nutritionresearchcenter.org/healthnews/farm-raised-fish-not-so-safe/.

12. http://www.whfoods.com/genpage.php?tname=george&dbid=96.

13. http://www.nrdc.org/health/effects/mercury/guide.asp.

14. http://www.veghealthguide.com/nuts-seeds/.

Chapter 11, Step 11: Train for Life

1. *Franklin's Merriam-Webster's Dictionary & Thesaurus*, 2004, s.v. "Intensity."

2. Ibid. "Intense."

Chapter 12, Step 12: Be a Revolution!

1. *Franklin Merriam-Webster's Dictionary & Thesaurus*, 2004, s.v. "Revolution."

2.   Ibid., s.v. "Radical."

3.   Ibid., s.v. "Extreme."

4.   Romans 12:2 New International Version.

5.   *Franklin Merriam-Webster's Dictionary & Thesaurus,* 2004, s.v. "Renew."

AUTHOR CONTACT

I am committed to inspiring those who want to be better, by empowering them to know their *wellth* and prosper in health so they can be their best. I passionately believe I am called to share this message with you, as well as with countless other dynamic, courageous individuals like you. I have a heart for helping people live a naturally drug-free, healthy life, with purpose and with passion.

I look forward to hearing from you.

To purchase books, for more information, or to schedule
Dr. Shannon to speak, please contact:

Dr. Shannon Subramanian

8002 S. 101st E. Avenue

Tulsa, OK 74133

www.drshannonknows.com

drshannon@drshannonknows.com

NOTES

NOTES

NOTES